# The Complete
# DASH Diet
## for Beginners

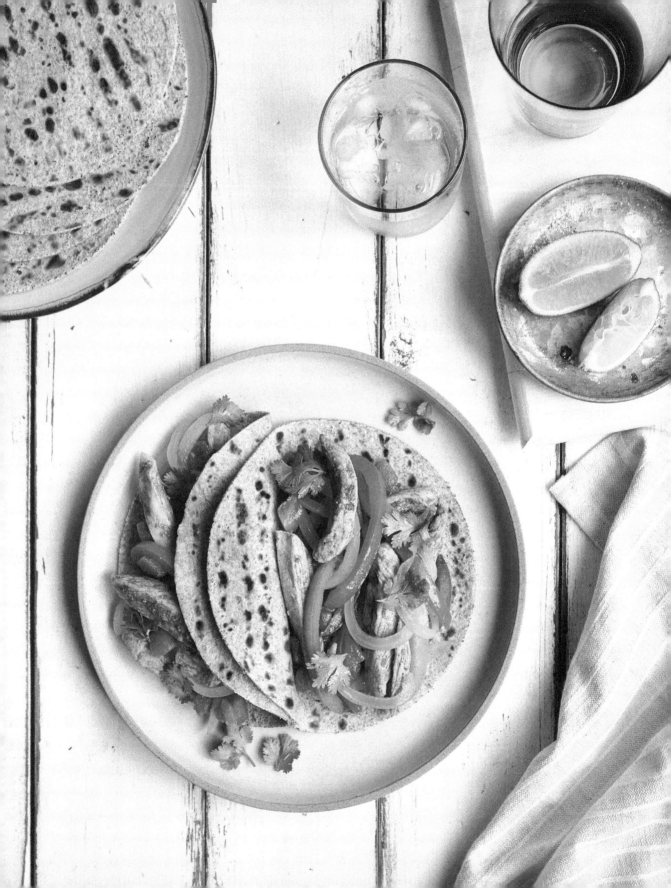

# The Complete
# DASH Diet
## for Beginners

### The Essential Guide to
### Lose Weight and Live Healthy

**JENNIFER KOSLO, PhD, RDN, CSSD**

ROCKRIDGE
PRESS

This book is dedicated
to my mother and father,
Erma and Walter.

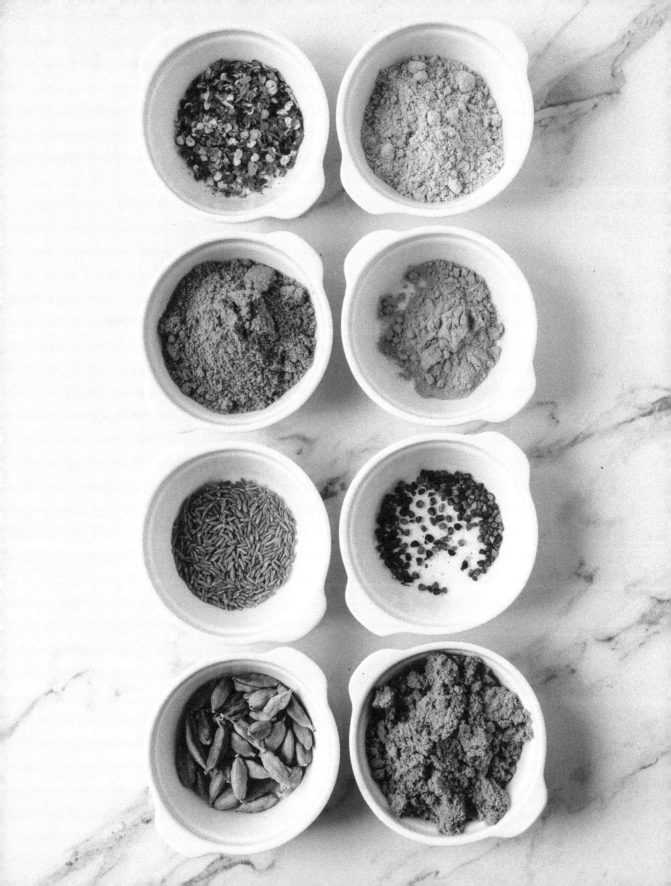

# Contents

*Introduction* viii

## PART ONE Living the DASH Diet

*one*   Dietary Approaches to Stop Hypertension  1

*two*   DASH in Five Steps  11

*three*   Week One Meal Plan & Recipes  23

*four*   Week Two Meal Plan & Recipes  41

## PART TWO Recipes for DASH Living

*five*   Breakfasts & Smoothies  61

*six*   Vegetarian & Vegan Mains  73

*seven*   Poultry & Seafood Mains  91

*eight*   Beef & Pork Mains  109

*nine*   Snacks, Sides & Desserts  121

*ten*   Broths, Condiments & Sauces  139

*Appendix A: The Dirty Dozen & The Clean Fifteen*  151

*Appendix B: Measurement Conversions*  152

*References*  153

*Resources*  154

*Recipe Index*  156

*Index*  158

# Introduction

**I often hear exclamations like** "I'm a believer!" from clients who have turned their health around by following the DASH diet. An acronym for Dietary Approaches to Stop Hypertension, the diet outlines an eating plan that is low in fat but rich in low-fat dairy foods, fruits, vegetables, whole grains, lean protein, beans, and nuts. It is designed to lower blood pressure and to help reduce the need for costly medications. Because DASH emphasizes consuming so many different kinds of healthy foods, many people find shedding pounds a welcomed side effect.

While not a magic bullet for everyone in pursuit of weight loss, the DASH diet is one that I personally trust and have recommended throughout my career as a registered dietitian nutritionist, as a cardiac rehab dietitian, and in my personal practice. I have seen firsthand how health can be transformed when I coach clients to fill their plates with foods recommended on the DASH diet, to watch their portions, and to exercise regularly. Without counting calories or feeling deprived, my clients have lost weight and have seen their blood pressure drop.

Unlike other untested eating plans, the DASH diet is one you can trust. Created by the National Heart, Lung, and Blood Institute (NHLBI), it is endorsed by the US government and backed by research from numerous clinical trials. For example, the DASH diet has again been ranked #1 by the *U.S. News & World Report* in the Best Diet for 2017 category. By the report's standards, to be considered top rated, a diet had to be relatively easy to follow, nutritious, safe, effective for weight loss, and protective against diabetes and heart disease. Compared with other diets, the DASH diet creates a well-rounded plan that does not focus on strict portion sizes, eliminating food groups, or gimmicks. Not obsessed with weight loss alone, the diet focuses on healthy choices—a stronger foundation for long-term success.

Designed with the beginner in mind, this book will be your handy all-in-one guide to starting the DASH diet today. Chapters 1 and 2 will give you a quick but solid understanding of the DASH diet, including an explanation of hypertension basics, simple guidelines for following the

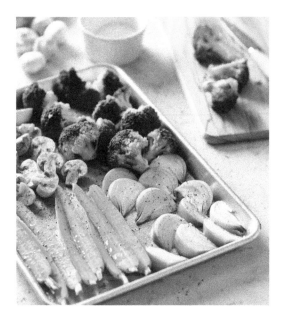
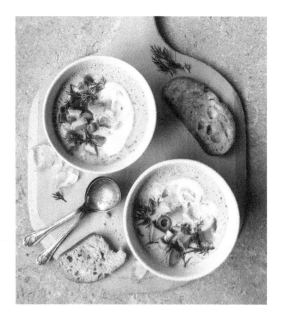

DASH diet, a table of what to eat when you are on the DASH diet, and practical steps to transition to a DASH lifestyle with ease. To make getting started even easier, there are two stand-alone seven-day meal plans with shopping lists, so you can get started right away. Importantly, the recipes include no more than five main ingredients, don't require expensive or hard-to-find items, and you don't need to be a chef to prepare them.

If you are reading this book, then you have already taken an important step by making your health, or the health of a loved one, a priority—congratulations! One of the biggest parts of becoming healthy is taking control and becoming informed. This book will make it easy for you to embrace a diet proven to lower blood pressure, cholesterol, and the risk for a number of chronic diseases. And you can start all this right now. Change your thinking about dieting, evolve from limiting yourself to thinking about what you can add to your diet, and what you can add to your life. Find your inner motivation, whether it is to be able to keep up with your grandchildren or to finally walk that half-marathon—harness your inner drive and make the commitment to optimize your health. If you stick with it and believe in yourself, you're going to reach your goal. Get ready to embrace the new you. I believe in you.

# PART ONE

# Living the DASH Diet

DASH is a flexible eating plan that encourages you to eat a wide variety of familiar whole foods, providing you with the nutrients you need to lower your blood pressure naturally. By learning to fill your plate with whole grains, vegetables, fruits, low-fat dairy products, fish, poultry, and legumes, you may see lower blood pressure in just two weeks. Besides weight loss, DASH offers other health benefits, too, including a lower risk of cancer, diabetes, heart disease, stroke, and osteoporosis. The DASH diet is mainly plant-based but is flexible and adaptable to your favorite foods, tastes, and lifestyle. Much more than a diet, DASH is a way of life that your whole family can follow to be healthy.

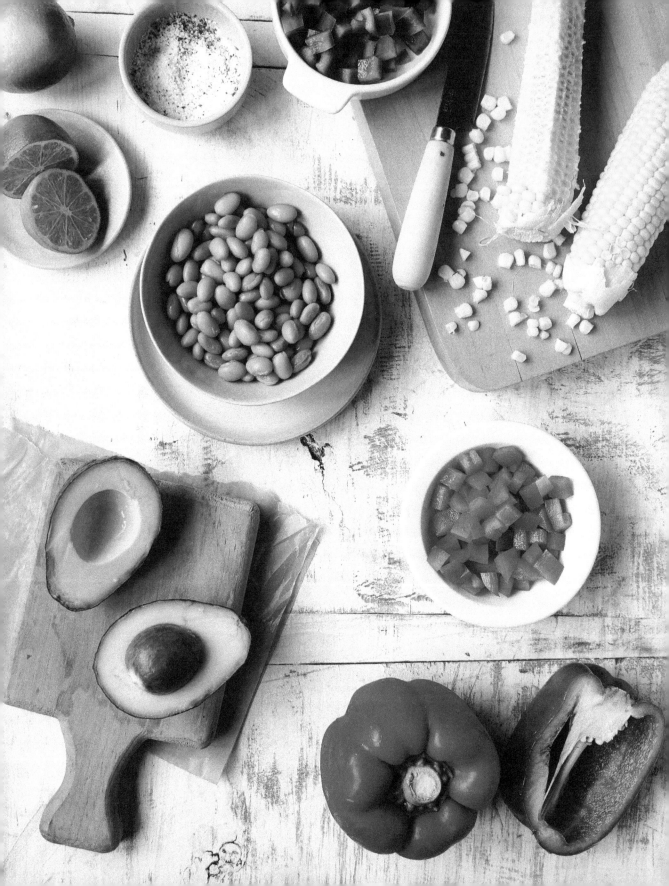

# one

# Dietary Approaches to Stop Hypertension

**Controlling hypertension** and improving your health involves creating a more balanced, healthier lifestyle overall. In this chapter, you will learn what high blood pressure is, gain an understanding of the condition's symptoms and risks, and learn how high blood pressure can harm your health. Guidelines for following the DASH diet will be presented along with simple, practical tips to help you with incorporating the diet into your lifestyle. Despite the fact that the original DASH-diet research was not designed for weight loss, new DASH research studies have focused on increasing the nutrient density of the diet and have shown even better results. The information, meal plans, and recipes in this book adhere to the latest research available.

If you suffer from high blood pressure and are currently taking medication to treat it, it is important to speak with your medical professional or a registered dietitian nutritionist before making any drastic changes to your diet. The DASH diet has been proven to lower blood pressure by several points in as little as two weeks, reducing or eliminating the need for first-line medication, however, results will vary. Do not stop taking your medication without your physician's approval, as this may put your health at an increased risk.

# Hypertension Basics

Each time your heart beats, blood is pumped through the arteries, veins, and blood vessels of your circulatory system—and the latter carries the blood throughout the body. Your blood pressure measurement takes into account both the amount of blood your heart pumps and the amount of resistance to the blood flow in your arteries. Narrow arteries increase resistance to blood flow, meaning that your heart has to work harder to deliver blood. The harder your heart has to work, the higher your blood pressure; this is a dangerous condition called *hypertension*. Over the long term, increased blood pressure can cause health issues, including heart disease.

The best way to know if you have high blood pressure is to have it checked and understand what the numbers mean. A blood pressure reading has a top number (systolic) and a bottom number (diastolic). The ranges are:

- Normal: Less than 120 over less than 80 (<120/<80)

- Prehypertension: 120–139 over 80–89

- Stage 1 high blood pressure (hypertension): 140–159 over 90–99

- Stage 2 high blood pressure (hypertension): 160 or higher over 100 or higher

- Hypertensive crisis (emergency care needed): higher than 180 over higher than 110

- High blood pressure in people over age 60: 150 and higher over 90 and higher

High blood pressure generally develops over many years, and it affects nearly everyone. It is known as "the silent killer" because you can have high blood pressure for years without any obvious symptoms. But even without symptoms, high blood pressure can cause damage to your arteries and blood vessels. And while blood pressure naturally increases as we age, there are several factors and conditions that can increase your risk for developing hypertension, including:

- Smoking

- Being overweight or obese

- Family history of high blood pressure

- Lack of physical activity

- A diet too high in salt

- A diet too low in potassium, calcium, and magnesium

- Drinking too much alcohol (more than two drinks a day for men, and more than one drink a day for women)

- Stress

- Being over 60 years of age

- Chronic kidney disease

- Race (African Americans, for example, are twice as likely as whites to have high blood pressure)

If left undetected or uncontrolled through treatment, high blood pressure can lead to heart attack, stroke, heart failure, kidney disease or failure, vision loss, sexual dysfunction, angina (chest pain), and peripheral artery disease (PAD). Your best protection is to have your blood pressure checked regularly, especially if you have one or more of the risk factors listed previously. Many pharmacies often have free blood-pressure-measurement machines at which you can obtain a reading in a matter of minutes. However, these do have limitations. The accuracy of such machines depends on several factors, like correct cuff size and proper use of the device. Speak with your doctor for advice on using public blood-pressure machines.

If you do have high blood pressure, the following is a list of the most common treatment recommendations:

- **Medications:** Known as antihypertensives, high-blood-pressure medications are available by prescription. There are a variety of classes of drugs, including diuretics, beta blockers, and ACE inhibitors among others. Your physician will work with you to prescribe the right medication for your individual condition.

- **Diet:** Following a well-balanced, low-salt diet—like the DASH eating plan—is likely to be part of your physician's lifestyle-change advice. Your health-care provider may also recommend you limit your alcohol consumption and stop smoking (if you do so).

*Eat more veggies, fruits, whole grains, lean protein, beans, and low-fat dairy products. Eat less sodium, fatty foods, red meat, and sugar. Drink alcohol in moderation.* When transitioning to the DASH diet, you want to focus on making healthy food and beverage choices from all five food groups, including fruits, vegetables, grains, protein foods, and dairy to get the nutrients you need.

- **Physical activity:** Physical activity can help you control your hypertension, manage your weight, strengthen your heart, and lower your stress levels. Additional information and tips for incorporating regular physical activity into your routine will be provided in chapter 2.

Understanding the effects of high blood pressure may make it easier for you to find your inner motivations, enabling you to make the lifestyle changes you need. Change is hard and can seem overwhelming at first, but by picking up this book you have already taken the first step. While there is no cure for high blood pressure, using medications as prescribed and making positive lifestyle changes can greatly enhance your life and reduce your risk of heart disease, stroke, and other chronic diseases.

# Guidelines for the DASH Diet

The DASH diet is rich in the minerals potassium, magnesium, and calcium, is high in fiber, and has a low content of sodium (salt) and saturated fat. Adding more of these nutrients will improve the electrolyte balance in the body, allowing it to excrete excess fluids whose presence contributes to high blood pressure. These nutrients also promote relaxation of the blood vessels, allowing blood to flow more freely, which in turn lowers blood pressure. Because these nutrients are often deficient in the standard American diet and in people who are overweight and obese, the DASH diet can help correct those deficiencies and help people from all walks of life feel better. The revised and latest DASH guidelines may also help promote weight loss, but incorporating regular physical activity will also be important in achieving this.

Because the DASH diet has no set foods, you can adapt your current diet to the DASH guidelines by doing the following:

**Eat more vegetables and fruits.** Fruits and vegetables are rich sources of potassium, magnesium, and fiber. "Eat the rainbow" and aim for a colorful mix of your favorite fresh fruits and vegetables each day. If you don't have access to fresh produce, use frozen and canned options without added salt.

*Focus on portion sizes and get the right amount of calories for you.* Visualize your plate each time you eat and fill half of it with veggies and fruits, ¼ with high-fiber whole grains, and ¼ with lean protein.

**Swap refined grains for whole grains.** Whole grains are major sources of slow-burning energy, are high in fiber, and are a rich source of important B vitamins. Choose whole-wheat bread over white and brown rice in place of white rice.

**Choose low-fat and nonfat dairy products.** Dairy products are major sources of calcium, vitamin D, and protein. Drink low-fat and nonfat milk with meals. Consume low-fat yogurts and cheese for snacks.

**Choose lean protein sources like fish, poultry, and beans.** Fish and poultry are rich sources of protein and magnesium. Beans are abundant sources of energy, magnesium, protein, and fiber. Remove the skin from poultry and cook fish and poultry by broiling, roasting, or poaching.

**Limit your intake of foods high in added sugars, like soda and candy.** Added sugars can contribute to weight gain and do not add any nutritive value to your diet. Limit sweets and added sugars to 9 teaspoons per day for men (150 calories, or 36 grams), and 6 teaspoons per day for women (100 calories, or 25 grams).

# WHAT TO EAT (AND NOT EAT) ON THE DASH DIET

| FOOD GROUP / ENJOY FREELY | EAT IN MODERATION (limited to 1 serving or fewer per day) | AVOID OR LIMIT |
|---|---|---|
| *dairy* Nonfat milk, 1% fat milk, low-fat, and nonfat cheese; low-fat and nonfat yogurt; low-fat and nonfat cottage cheese; low-fat and nonfat ricotta cheese; nonfat cream cheese; nonfat sour cream | 2% fat milk (8 ounces), low-fat cream cheese (1 tablespoon), low-fat sour cream (1 tablespoon) | Whole milk, full-fat cheese, regular sour cream, regular cream cheese, full-fat yogurt |
| *fruits* Citrus, berries, bananas, grapes, melons, pineapple, mangoes, peaches, apricots, apples, pears, plums, kiwi | Avocado (½), dried fruit (¼ cup) | None |
| *grains* Whole-wheat and whole-grain breads, whole-grain breakfast cereals, wheat germ, brown rice, bulgur, whole-wheat couscous, quinoa, oatmeal | White bread (1 slice), white pasta (½ cup cooked), white rice (½ cup cooked) | Sugar-filled breakfast cereals, donuts, pastries, cakes, cookies, pies |
| *fats and oils* Canola oil, olive oil, vegetable oils | Butter (1 teaspoon), mayonnaise (1 tablespoon), salad dressing (1 tablespoon) | Coconut oil, palm oil, lard, solid margarine |
| *proteins* Lean poultry, fish, eggs, beans, legumes, tofu | Nuts and seeds (⅓ cup of nuts, 2 tablespoons seeds, 2 tablespoons nut butter), red meat (6 ounces or fewer) | Bacon, sausage, hot dogs, luncheon meats, and smoked, cured, or pickled foods |
| *vegetables* Tomatoes, carrots, summer squash, broccoli, leafy greens, mushrooms, green beans, cabbage, cauliflower, asparagus, Brussels sprouts, onions | Winter squash (½ cup), corn (½ cup), green peas (⅔ cup) | None |

**Limit your intake of foods high in saturated fats like fatty meats, full-fat dairy, and oils such as coconut and palm oils.** The DASH study used a 2,000-calorie eating plan with daily nutrient goals that included 27 percent of total calories as fat (that's with fat for cooking and as added to foods). To make things easy, cook with vegetable oils, choose red meat only once weekly, and limit full-fat dairy products to a single serving per day.

**Choose and prepare foods with less salt and sodium.** Keep the saltshaker off the table and become creative with herbs, spices, lemon, lime, vinegar, and salt-free seasoning blends. And because most of the sodium we eat comes from processed foods, be sure to read food labels to check sodium levels, aiming for foods with 5 percent or less of the daily value of sodium.

The DASH diet recommends a dietary pattern that focuses on the number of daily servings from various food groups. The number of servings depends on your individual calorie needs. Your calorie level depends on your age, gender, and how active you are. If you want to maintain your current weight, you should take in only as many calories as you burn by being physically active. If you want to lose weight, eat fewer calories than you burn or increase your activity level to burn more calories than you eat.

For a 2,000-calorie diet, the following servings are recommended each day: 2 to 2½ cups of fruits; 2 to 2½ cups of vegetables; 6 to 8 (1-ounce) servings of whole grains; 6 ounces or fewer of meats, fish, and poultry;

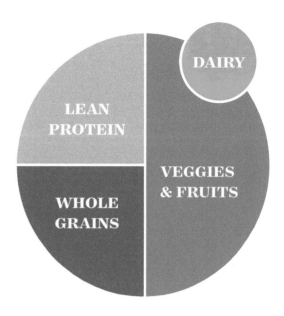

2 to 3 cups per day of nonfat or low-fat milk; and 2 to 3 teaspoons of oils. In addition, DASH recommends 4 to 5 servings per week of nuts, seeds, and legumes.

To make it easy to meet these goals, simply visualize your plate and at each meal aim to fill half of it with vegetables and fruits, a quarter with lean protein, and the last quarter with whole grains. You should also have 1 serving of nonfat or low-fat dairy. To keep calories and portions in check, always choose a 9-inch plate.

While the DASH diet has two levels of sodium—2,300 milligrams and 1,500 milligrams—the recipes in this book will be very low in sodium and appropriate for the lowest sodium level. Remember that fruits and vegetables are naturally low in sodium, so DASH makes it easier to eat less of it. Keep in mind: The less sodium you eat, the more you may be able to lower your blood pressure.

# DASH-FRIENDLY DRINKS

If drinking soda and juice is a daily habit, you may at first find it difficult to go without them, especially if you're not fond of plain water. Start by tapering yourself off: Mix half your normal serving of soda or juice with sparking water and add extra ice. You'll still get the sweetness you're craving with a healthy dose of the water your body needs. It's also easy to infuse your water with fruits, vegetables, or herbs to make it more appealing to drink. For best results, gently squeeze citrus, cube melons, and crush berries before inserting into a bottle; herbs should be crushed, not chopped. Then fill your bottle with water, shake, and let steep for a few minutes (or overnight in the refrigerator) before consuming. These are my favorite combinations: strawberry and blueberry, lemon and cucumber, lemon and lime, orange and raspberry, lemon and basil, cucumber and mint, lavender and orange.

If you really want to add nutrients to your diet, why not swap your soda for a glass of milk? The DASH diet recommends at least three servings of dairy products each day, as dairy products are rich in calcium, an important nutrient involved in blood-pressure regulation. Even better, clinical trials have shown that the milk you consume doesn't have to be nonfat, giving you the freedom to choose 1 or 2%t milk without losing the positive health benefits.

How does alcohol fit in? It's important to understand that too much alcohol can elevate blood pressure. You don't need to eliminate alcohol if it is part of your routine, but you will need to keep portions in check. Moderate drinking for a male is two drinks per day, and for a woman it is one drink a day. A drink is considered 12 ounces of beer, 5 ounces of wine, or 1½ ounces of liquor. To reap alcohol's heart-healthy benefits, choose red wines with a dry flavor profile (like Cabernets), which are higher in flavonoids (cardio-protective plant antioxidants). As a general rule, the sweeter the wine, the lower its flavonoid levels.

# DASH and Diabetes

A healthy diet is an essential tool for people managing type 2 diabetes. While there are many plans to choose from, the DASH eating plan is an excellent choice. Ranked by the *U.S. News & World Report* as the #1 best diet for managing type 2 diabetes, the improved DASH diet can promote weight loss—effectively lowering both A1C levels (a test measuring your average blood sugar over the last three months) and fasting blood-glucose levels (your glucose level when you haven't had anything to eat for a prolonged length of time). By eliminating the empty carbohydrates and starchy foods from your diet, as is done in the revised version of DASH, you can avoid the simple sugars that the body easily absorbs and quickly sends into the bloodstream, causing insulin levels to spike. If you have type 2 diabetes and currently eat a more typical American diet, keep the following cautions in mind when transitioning to the DASH diet:

**Up your carbs and mind your starch.** Increase the amount of low-carbohydrate vegetables you eat while keeping portions of starchy vegetables in check. Vegetables low in carbohydrates—like zucchini, cauliflower, mushrooms, and leafy greens—will not cause a spike in blood sugar and can be eaten freely. Starchy vegetables like corn, potatoes, and winter squash, which are all nutritious, are high in carbohydrates and

*Become label literate.* Use nutrition-information labels and ingredients lists to help you make healthy choices by finding the amounts of saturated fats, sodium, and added sugars in the foods and beverages you choose.

could contribute to a rise in blood sugar. To include these nutritious veggies, simply use them in place of grains at meals.

**Remember your grains.** The DASH diet calls for two additional 1-ounce servings of grains. To prevent a rise in blood sugar, choose high-fiber whole grains like brown rice or rolled oats, pairing them with protein and healthy fats, as the fiber, protein, and fat will slow the digestion of these grains, providing an even release of energy.

**Drink your milk.** The DASH diet recommends three servings per day of milk and dairy products. Choose nonfat or low-fat milk and remember to count it as part of your meal plan. One cup of nonfat milk provides about 12 grams of carbohydrates, but it also contains important vitamins and minerals and is a good source of protein. Just remember to stick to standard 8-ounce portion sizes when you drink milk because the calories and carbohydrates can add up when you have too much.

# Benefits to Look Forward To

Anyone who makes a change to their diet will experience the symptoms of that change. The experience will be different for everyone because people come to the DASH diet from unique starting points in terms of diet quality and composition. However, knowing that your mind and body need to adjust to change will help you keep moving forward.

## What to Expect in the Short Term

If you are used to following a more standard American diet, you may find that your transition to the DASH eating plan will result in unexpected side effects, both positive and negative ones. Drastically reducing the amount of salt, fat, sugar, and refined carbohydrates could lead to cravings for the foods you initially cut from your diet. Remember, these cravings are only temporary, and once your body gets used to a lower intake, your palate will change and you will no longer experience cravings. Be prepared for when cravings strike and keep your kitchen stocked with healthy snacks like fresh fruits and vegetables. On the positive side, cutting out sources of empty calories may lead to a welcome loss of weight, especially if you combine the DASH diet with a regular exercise program.

## What to Expect in the Long Term

Depending on how closely you follow the DASH eating pattern, you may find your blood-pressure readings decrease by several points in just two weeks. In the long term, following the DASH diet will reduce your risk of cancer, lower your risk for metabolic syndrome, lower your risk for type 2 diabetes, decrease your heart-disease risk, and, if you are overweight, help you shed the pounds. You may also find you sleep better, your digestion could improve, and you could experience more energy.

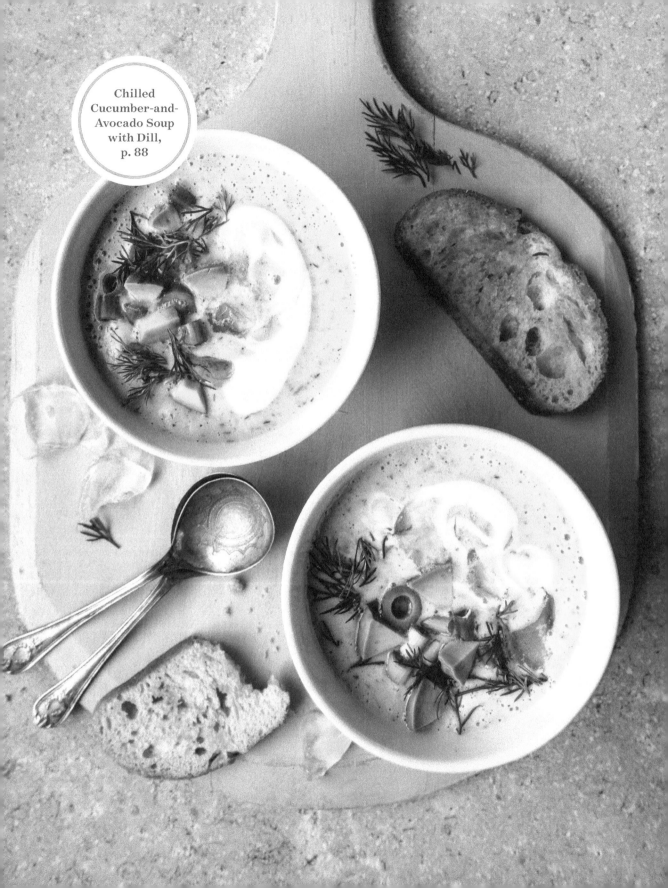

Chilled
Cucumber-and-
Avocado Soup
with Dill,
p. 88

# *two*

# DASH in Five Steps

**The DASH eating plan requires no special foods** and doesn't have hard-to-follow rules. It simply calls for a certain number of daily servings from various food groups. That said, any type of dietary change is hard and can feel daunting at first. Challenges are bound to appear along the way. It's important to remember that your transition to the DASH eating style will happen gradually, not all at once, and it is okay to take it slow, one step at a time. Your ultimate goal is to establish new eating habits that can be sustained for a lifetime. To give you time to get used to your new eating behaviors, some experts suggest making just one change each week. The following sections provide an easy step-by-step guide to get you started on your DASH eating plan, helping your transition be as smooth as possible.

# Step 1: Clean Out Your Pantry

DASH is more than a diet. The ultimate goal is starting a new life and embarking on a sustainable, enjoyable, healthy eating pattern—and it all starts in the kitchen. In order to be successful with DASH you have to set yourself up for success, which means you need to surround yourself with nutritious foods and purge the foods that are holding you back. If a food or drink that isn't conducive to your goals is conveniently near, either you or someone you love will eventually eat it. A pantry clean-out removes the foods that trigger poor eating behaviors and replaces them with health-promoting foods. This step is essential, as it makes food decisions foolproof, helping you stay in control and on track.

While DASH is a healthy eating pattern recommended for everyone, young and old, you may have household members who aren't quite ready to give up the ice cream and chips, or maybe you have kids who run from fruits and vegetables. If your family isn't ready to get on board with your healthy eating plan, don't get frustrated or stressed. Avoid pushing the issue; simply start being a role model and you might be surprised how others start to follow suit once they see how great you feel. If you are worried about the temptation of unhealthy foods, create a designated shelf in your pantry or in a cupboard— not on the countertop or front-row in the refrigerator—for family-member treats.

*Change gradually.* Transition your diet to the DASH eating plan over a couple of weeks to give yourself a chance to adjust and make the changes a part of your daily routine. For example, add a serving of vegetables at lunch one day and at dinner the next day, and add fruits at one meal or as a snack.

Keeping trigger foods out of sight will make them relatively easy to forget about.

Next you will want to take stock of the items you currently have in your pantry, refrigerator, and freezer. Make note of the foods you currently eat that are processed. Read the ingredients labels and plan to donate or use up all items high in salt, sugar, and saturated fat. Use the following list of guidelines to get started on your pantry clean-out:

1. **Donate or toss out pre-prepared foods.** "Complete" meals like seasoning mixes for hamburgers, preseasoned rice mixes, and boxed macaroni and cheese are all high in salt, added fats, and preservatives. Check your canned soups, as most are very high in sodium and should be used up or donated.

2. **Read cereal labels for sugar content.** If you have breakfast cereals, read the nutrition facts panel, and if your cereal contains more than 4 to 6 grams of sugar per serving, which is about 1 to 1½ teaspoons of sugar, donate it or toss it out.

3. **Sort through your snacks.** If they're processed—think crackers, potato chips, cookies, cakes, or candy—donate them or just toss them out. Treats like this can be donated to organizations that support our overseas military personnel by creating care packages with donated items.

4. **Next, search your freezer.** After finishing with your pantry, it's time for the freezer. The majority of frozen dinners are high in sodium, calories, and unhealthy fats while being low in fiber, whole grains, and vegetables. They generally are poor food choices. If you have vegetables in sauces, these will also be high in sodium. Donate or toss out.

5. **Make note of what you have.** Lastly, take a refrigerator inventory. If you have smoked meats, bacon, sausage, pickled foods, hot dogs, or lunch meat, again, donate or toss.

While purging will be painful and you may experience feelings of resentment, if the food isn't going to help you reach your goals, you don't need it. Now that you have cleaned your pantry, it is time to fill it up. Next you will learn how to restock with health-promoting choices that won't break your budget.

# Step 2: Go Shopping

After you finish cleaning out your pantry, it's time to restock the pantry, refrigerator, and freezer with DASH-appropriate foods.

This section will provide general pantry guidelines and the next chapter will provide separate pantry lists for the two weekly meal plans. And while it is not necessary to purchase organic, free-range, or locally grown produce, two of the Environmental Working Group's annual lists—The Dirty Dozen and the Clean Fifteen—will be provided in Appendix A (page 151). Consider reviewing the list, making note of any foods there that you eat frequently, and, as budget allows, explore purchasing organic for those foods only. Other ways to stay within budget are to buy store brand rather than name brand products. Just check the ingredients list to confirm that the products are comparable. The Resources section (page 154) lists some chains that carry their own brand of budget-friendly products.

The following list of pantry staples includes items that are good to keep on hand so you can prepare meals with little to no planning. The list includes basic ingredients that are used often in recipes and, with the exception of the fresh ingredients, are fairly inexpensive and have a long shelf life. Your personal list will take shape as you begin to cook on a regular basis according to your personal tastes. One important note is that while many people think frozen produce is not as nutritious as fresh, it is in fact often *more* nutritious, since the food is processed immediately after harvesting, retaining high levels of nutrients. Frozen produce won't spoil. And the best part is that frozen produce is inexpensive, meaning that using it cuts down on food waste.

# DON'T FORGET SELF-CARE

Starting a new diet seems to bring out the self-critic in people, that little inner voice that berates you for a lack of willpower or makes you feel guilty about your food choices. If this sounds familiar, you aren't alone. Research has shown that self-compassion is often the missing ingredient in attempts to start healthy eating habits. Self-compassion has the power to make or break your success at eating well. The more understanding and forgiving we are of ourselves, the more motivated we are to do what we need to do to take care of ourselves.

According to self-compassion researcher Kristin Neff, PhD, self-compassion consists of three main components:

*Self-kindness* Instead of criticizing yourself, be kind and understanding of yourself in instances of failure.

*Common humanity* Recognize you are not alone.

*Mindfulness* Keep thoughts and feelings in a balanced awareness, neither over-identifying with them or ignoring them.

The following are five ways you can practice self-compassion:

1. *Give up black-and-white thinking.* Healthy eating is flexible and can include a wide variety of choices, some healthier than others. Give yourself permission to mindfully enjoy a small portion of your favorite food. This helps prevent feelings of deprivation and helps avoid over-eating later.

2. *Become aware of self-talk.* Our thoughts create our reality. Notice how often your inner chatter admonishes you for eating too much or not eating what you should have. Talk to yourself in a kind and under-standing way, as you would to a very good friend.

3. *Ask for what you want and need.* Do you need your partner to help you with the shopping? Do you need your partner to watch the kids so you can get a walk in? Be your own advocate.

**4.** *Practice self-compassion through writing*. When you feel bad about yourself, write yourself a letter about the issue from the perspective of a friend who knows you and loves you unconditionally. How would your friend let you know you are human and have both strengths and weaknesses?

**5.** *Finish on a positive note.* End your day reflecting on three things that you did well. Reflecting on successes rather than missteps will help shift your mind to more compassionate thoughts.

By adopting a loving, curious, open, and forgiving attitude toward yourself, you can foster a healthy relationship with eating and food, opening the door to improved health and long-term happiness.

One final note: Use this list as a general guide for what items are good to keep on hand, but please don't feel like you have to go out and purchase all of these items before you begin to cook. Buy one or two new items each week until you have a well-stocked kitchen, and remember to always work within your budget.

**Pantry Basics:** Canned beans, dry lentils, canned no-salt diced tomatoes, low-sodium vegetables, low-sodium chicken broth, rolled oats, steel-cut oats, whole-wheat flour, brown rice, whole-grain pasta, unsalted nuts, natural peanut butter, flavored vinegars, and herbs and spices including black pepper, basil, cumin, garlic, onion, oregano, thyme, cinnamon.

**Vegetables:** Frozen spinach, frozen peas, frozen broccoli, frozen cauliflower, fresh leafy greens, tomatoes, mushrooms, summer squash, carrots, cabbage, broccoli, onions, sweet potatoes.

**Proteins:** Frozen skinless boneless chicken breasts, frozen boneless fish fillets, frozen shrimp, eggs, lean ground beef, lean ground turkey.

**Fruit:** Apples, bananas, citrus, avocado, frozen berries.

**Dairy:** Low-fat milk of choice (dairy, soy), nonfat or low-fat Greek yogurt, low-fat shredded cheese, Parmesan cheese.

**Fats and Oils:** Olive oil, canola oil, soft margarine.

# Step 3: Set Up Your Kitchen

Just as you need to select the ingredients you know you will use, select kitchen equipment you are comfortable with. The recipes in this book require a minimum amount of equipment, while still taking advantage of labor-saving devices. Make your kitchen a friendly, welcoming, organized place. Your time in the kitchen should be pleasant and it should be easy for you to prep and prepare meals. The following two lists include essential equipment and nice-to-have equipment.

## Essential Equipment

This list of essential equipment includes items needed for daily cooking, aimed at the beginner cook:

**Nonstick skillet or frying pan with lid.** A good nonstick skillet is indispensable, making it easy to brown, fry, and sauté. Choose a size that works for you according to the number of people in your household.

**A small and a large pot, with lids.** A small and a large saucepan will be used in this book to prepare sauces, soups, and stews. Choosing ones with a nonstick coating will make clean up easy and won't require a lot of oil when using. Nontoxic eco-friendly options include glass, ceramic, stainless steel, and green nonstick cookware.

**Baking dishes.** Glass or metal baking dishes are used for roasting meats and preparing casserole-type dishes. They are even useful for serving straight from the oven to the table and can be used to store leftovers.

**Rimmed 9-by-13-inch baking sheet.** A baking sheet with a 1-inch rim is designed to catch juices from roasting vegetables, meats, fish, and poultry. Choose from metal or silicone.

**Knives.** The two most important knives for efficient prep in the kitchen are a good-quality chef's knife for larger items, like meats, and a paring knife for fruits, vegetables, and herbs.

**Cutting boards.** A wooden cutting board will be easy on kitchen knives, keeping them sharp for longer. Dedicated cutting boards are ideal—one for fresh vegetables and fruits, one for meats—but this isn't always practical on a tight budget. If you are using one cutting board, be sure to avoid cross-contamination by sanitizing your board after working with raw meats and seafood.

**Assorted mixing bowls.** Look for durable nesting bowls that can handle large and small volumes. Look for bowls with lids, which can be used for storing leftovers.

**Blender.** A basic blender is needed to make smoothies and can also take the place of a food processor for puréeing soups and beans. Try to purchase one with at least

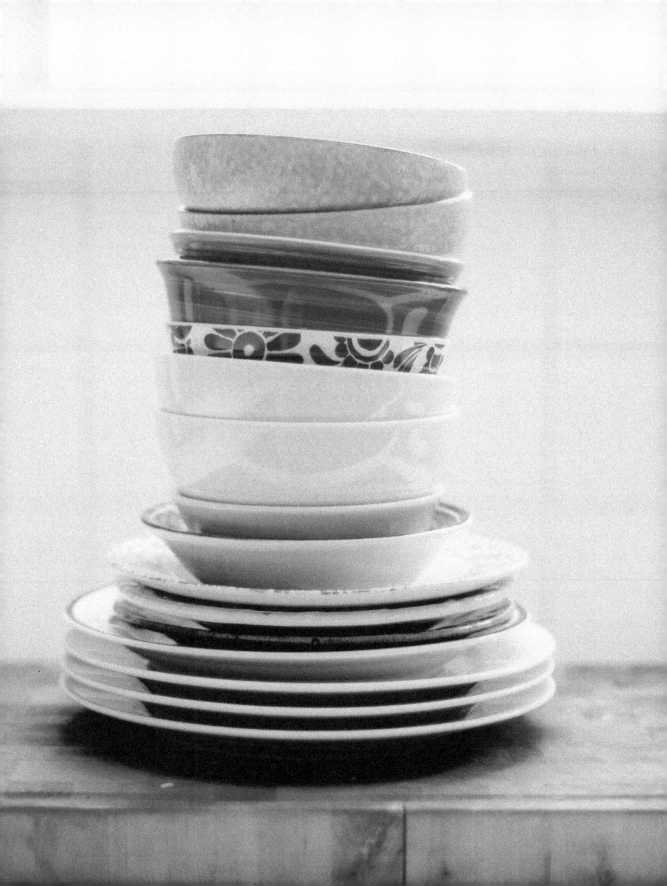

450 watts of power so you have the flexibility you need to effortlessly process a variety of ingredients.

**Other tools.** Other kitchen necessities you should have on hand include: a slotted spoon, spatula, wooden spoon, whisk, ladle, can opener, colander, measuring cups and spoons, timer, meat thermometer, vegetable peeler, oven mitts, pot holder, and kitchen towels.

## Nice-to-Have Equipment

**Food processor.** A food processor is nice to have for chopping, slicing, grating, dicing, and puréeing a variety of ingredients including nuts, beans, soups, vegetables, and grains. Food processors are similar to blenders but they have interchangeable blades and discs rather than a fixed blade.

**Spiralizer.** A spiralizer turns fresh veggies into faux noodles. Most models are about the size of a large toaster and function like a giant pencil sharpener. Spiralizing veggies and using them in place of pasta is a great way to boost your intake of vegetables while cutting back on calories.

**Slow cooker.** A slow cooker has many advantages and is a great way to save time while preparing a nutritious meal. Slow cookers can be used for breakfast casseroles, steel-cut oats, soups, stews, roasts, and grains.

# Step 4: Plan Your Meals

When it comes to eating well, meal planning is one of the easiest things you can do to set yourself up for success. Meal planning has no set rules and takes very little time, yet using a meal plan saves you money, frees up your time, cuts down on food waste, and prevents those "What's for dinner?" moments, which create temptations for convenience foods or ordering takeout.

There are a number of ways to approach meal planning—after practicing just a few times, you'll begin to find what works for you and your family. To help you get started, the next chapter offers two stand-alone seven-day meal plans with shopping lists for you to use right away. You can even customize the meal plans by interchanging any of the recipes within meal categories, as each is created to be budget friendly, quick to prepare, and DASH friendly.

To successfully integrate meal planning into your life, here is a step-by-step guide with some of the basics, so you can meal plan with a purpose:

**Set aside a regular time to meal plan.** It may seem obvious, but as with any goal, the first step is making the commitment. Choose a day that works for you, and involve those who eat with you by asking what they do and don't like to eat. Then, grab a pad of paper, a pen, this cookbook, and get inspired.

**Decide how many meals you are going to prepare for the week.** Take a few moments to think about your schedule for the next week and how many meals you have time to prepare. You will also want to consider your grocery budget, current sales, and what types of produce are in season.

**Pick your recipes.** Plan out all three meals (breakfast, lunch, and dinner) and select recipes with common ingredients to minimize how much you have to buy. Choose recipes that will help you meet your daily goals for the day. Note how many servings a recipe yields so you can repurpose meals and make use of leftovers.

**Before creating your shopping list, do a pantry, refrigerator, and freezer review.** Once you have your recipes and list of ingredients, do a pantry, refrigerator, and freezer review, and then create your list.

**Shop strategically.** Before you shop, check local flyers and coupon ads to take advantage of sales.

**Cook perishables first.** Designate one day as a cooking day and prepare meals in advance that reheat well, using perishables first. Prep ingredients for meals later in the week so that you have them ready to go when it's mealtime.

Once you have done meal planning and realized its time- and money-saving benefits—not to mention your new appetite for healthy meals—you'll never want to return to the stress and expense of not knowing what's for dinner.

*Treat meat as part of the meal instead of the focus.* If you usually eat large portions of meat, cut them back with the aim to reduce your consumption in half for a couple of days. Have two or more meatless meals each week. Try stir-fries, which have less meat but more vegetables, grains, and beans.

# Step 5: Get Fit and Active

To get the most benefit from the DASH diet, especially if you want to lose weight, you must incorporate regular physical activity into your daily routine. A physically active lifestyle is essential for lowering blood pressure, reducing your risk for heart disease, strengthening your muscles, and lowering stress levels. However, if it's been a while since you have been active, or you have recently been diagnosed with heart disease or diabetes—or have other co-morbidities like kidney disease, or are a male over the age of 40 or a female over the age of 50—it is important you obtain medical clearance from a physician before starting an exercise program.

The 2008 Physical Activity Guidelines for Americans recommends 150 minutes of moderate-intensity aerobic activity per week (such as 30 minutes of walking 5 days a week), muscle-strengthening activities on 2 or more days of the week, and a regular program of stretching.

*Use fruit for desserts and snacks.* Fruits do not contain sodium and have negligible amounts of fat (except for avocado). Choose them in place of cookies and refined treats for snacks and desserts. Try topping low-fat Greek yogurt with fresh berries to boost your intake of both dairy and fruits.

## Cardiovascular Exercise

Cardiovascular exercises are activities that work your heart and lungs and, as a result, increase your heart rate and breathing. Examples are walking, jogging, swimming, raking leaves, dancing, and playing tennis. Cardiovascular activities will make it easier for you to walk farther and complete everyday activities such as gardening, shopping, or housework with more ease. Brisk walking is probably one of the best ways to get active. It can be done anywhere and doesn't require any fancy equipment. You can also break up your 30 minutes into 10-minute pieces throughout the day, such as a 10-minute walk before breakfast, 10 minutes at lunch, and 10 minutes before dinner.

## Strength Training

Strength exercises build and maintain muscle. Even very small changes in muscle strength can make a real difference in your ability to perform everyday activities like carrying groceries, lifting a grandchild,

or doing housework. To build strength, you need to push or pull weight, and your bodyweight is all that you need to work all of your major muscle groups. You can also use weights, resistance bands, or common objects from your home. Remember to always include warm-up and cool-down exercises. You can work all of your major muscle groups at home using this sample bodyweight exercise routine:

1.  10 bodyweight squats

2.  10 pushups

3.  10 dumbbell rows (using a gallon milk jug or dumbbell)

4.  10 walking lunges

## Stretching

The older we get, the more likely we are to experience tight muscles, which can throw off our posture or make us prone to injuries. Stretching elongates the muscles around joints, which helps increase range of motion and in turn helps avoid injury. Stretching also reduces stress, improves mood, and generally makes you feel better. In terms of how often you should stretch, daily is ideal—but you can also do it when your muscles feel tight or your body feels off. Here are a couple of safe and effective stretches you can try:

**Quad pull.** This stretches your thighs and improves flexibility. Stand with your feet together and arms at your sides. Put your right hand on a wall or table for support, then balance on your right leg and bend your left knee back, bringing up your left foot until you can grab your ankle with your left hand. Take five deep breaths. Then switch sides and repeat.

**Arm opener.** This stretches your arms, chest, and shoulders. Stand with your feet comfortably apart. Take your hands and interlace them behind your tailbone with your knuckles down. Looking straight ahead, drive your arms up and away from your tailbone until you feel a comfortable stretch. Take five deep breaths and relax.

## One Day at a Time

Take the pressure off and start with a few DASH meals per week, making use of the sample menus provided in the next chapter. Focus on the DASH foods you already eat. When a meal or snack works, recycle and repeat your success! It's also important to include some type of daily stress-relieving activity—such as reading, yoga, or meditation—and to be certain you regularly get seven to eight hours of sleep. Too much stress and lack of sleep will undermine your efforts by increasing hunger and hormones like cortisol (which causes your body to store fat). Remember to keep things in perspective and celebrate every success—big or small—as you transition to a healthier you.

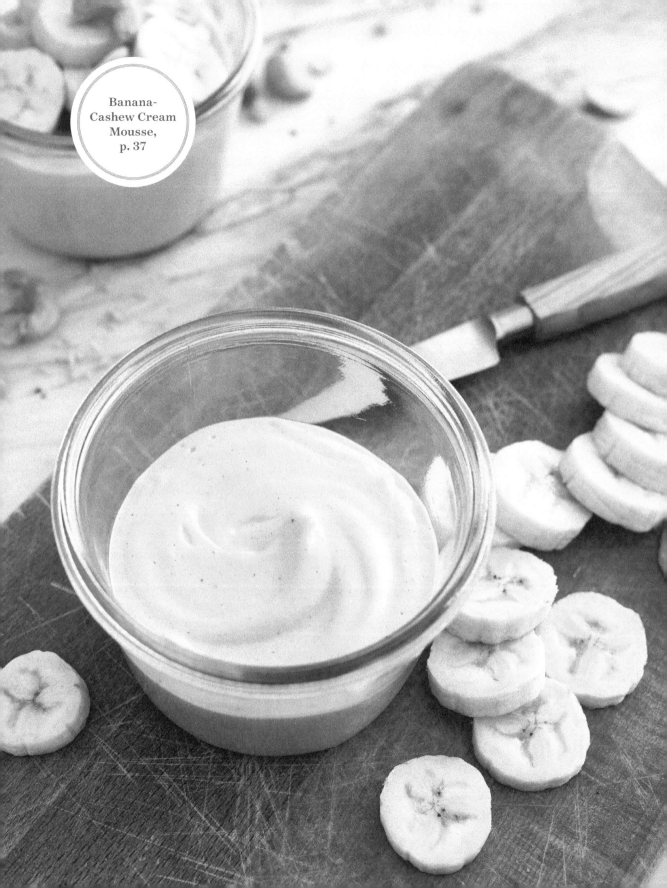

Banana-
Cashew Cream
Mousse,
p. 37

# *three*

# **Week One Meal Plan & Recipes**

**Now that you're familiar with the DASH diet** and understand that it emphasizes eating low-sodium foods that are rich in potassium, magnesium, and calcium—nutrients that lower blood pressure—it's time to start incorporating DASH into your daily mealtime routine.

To help you get started, in this chapter and chapter 4, I have provided two, seven-day meal plans that conform to the DASH diet. They are written for a single person, so if you are cooking for more than one, you will need to multiply the shopping lists and recipes. A very basic pantry list is also provided.

The recipes needed to prepare the meals in the meal plans are included in this chapter. The recipes will be grouped together by meal and appear in the meal plan's order of appearance. Not all meals will require recipes and instead suggestions will be made on what to eat so that you can use these menus as a basis for your own healthy meal planning. If a suggested meal or snack option doesn't appeal to you, simply make a DASH-friendly substitute using the recipes in this book. Remember that on some days you may eat a few more or less recommended servings of a particular food group. That's okay as long as the average for the week is close to the recommendations. The exception is sodium. Try to stay within the daily limit for sodium (1,500 milligrams) as much as possible.

# WEEK ONE SHOPPING LIST

This list outlines everything you need to make all the recipes for the week for one person to follow the plan.

## PANTRY LIST

- ☐ Almonds, unsalted
- ☐ Cooking spray, nonstick
- ☐ Garlic
- ☐ Olive oil
- ☐ Onions
- ☐ Peanut butter, unsalted
- ☐ Pepper
- ☐ Rolled oats
- ☐ Salt

## REFRIGERATED STAPLES

- ☐ Fruit, fresh
- ☐ Milk, nonfat or low-fat
- ☐ Salad greens

## FRESH PRODUCE

- ☐ Asparagus (1 bunch)
- ☐ Bananas (2)
- ☐ Brussels sprouts (14)
- ☐ Carrots (1 cup)
- ☐ Lemon (1)
- ☐ Mushrooms (1 cup)
- ☐ Onion, small (1)
- ☐ Spinach (8 cups)

*Optional for toppings*
- ☐ Avocado (1)
- ☐ Parsley (1 bunch)
- ☐ Rosemary (1 bunch)
- ☐ Tomato (1)

## OILS, VINEGARS & CONDIMENTS

- ☐ Lemon juice
- ☐ Mustard, Dijon
- ☐ Mustard, yellow
- ☐ Olive oil
- ☐ Vinegar, cider

## DRY GOODS

- ☐ Bread, whole-grain (1 loaf)
- ☐ Cashews (½ cup)
- ☐ Sugar

*Optional topping*
- ☐ Walnuts, chopped

## CANNED & BOTTLED GOODS

- ☐ Chickpeas (1 [15-ounce] can)
- ☐ Orange juice, 100 percent (¼ cup)
- ☐ Soy sauce, reduced-sodium

## DAIRY & EGGS

- ☐ Cheese, Parmesan, grated (¼ cup)
- ☐ Eggs (6)
- ☐ Milk, nonfat or low-fat (1½ cups)
- ☐ Yogurt, Greek, nonfat or low-fat, plain or flavored (3½ cups)
- ☐ String cheese, low-fat (1 pack)

## MEAT & SEAFOOD, PLUS MEAT ALTERNATIVES

- ☐ Beef, sirloin, boneless (½ pound)
- ☐ Flounder (2 [6-ounce] fillets)
- ☐ Pork, tenderloin (1 pound)
- ☐ Salmon (2 [5-ounce] fillets)
- ☐ Tofu, firm (8 ounces)

## FREEZER

- ☐ Cranberries (12 ounces)
- ☐ Peaches (2 cups)
- ☐ Pineapple (¼ cup)
- ☐ Spinach (1 cup)
- ☐ Stir-fry vegetables (3 cups)

## SEASONINGS & FLAVORINGS

- ☐ Chives, dried
- ☐ Cinnamon
- ☐ Cornstarch
- ☐ Cumin, dried
- ☐ Dill, dried
- ☐ Garlic, powder
- ☐ Nutmeg
- ☐ Paprika
- ☐ Rosemary, dried
- ☐ Tarragon, dried
- ☐ Vanilla extract

# WEEK ONE MENU

| | MONDAY | TUESDAY | WEDNESDAY |
|---|---|---|---|
| *breakfast* | Microwave Quiche in a Mug | 1 cup oatmeal topped with 1 tablespoon almonds, with 1 cup nonfat milk, 1 cup blueberries | Peaches and Greens Smoothie |
| *snack* | 1 apple, 1 cup low-fat Greek yogurt (flavored or plain) | Carrot-Cake Smoothie | 1 low-fat string cheese, ½ cup baby carrots |
| *lunch* | Southwest Tofu Scramble | Leftover Lemon-Parsley Baked Flounder and Brussels Sprouts | Leftover Baked Chickpea-and-Rosemary Omelet |
| *snack* | 1 banana, ¼ cup almonds | Carrot-Cake Smoothie | 1 apple, ¼ cup almonds |
| *dinner* | Lemon-Parsley Baked Flounder and Brussels Sprouts | Baked Chickpea-and-Rosemary Omelet plus side salad | Easy Roast Salmon with Roasted Asparagus |

| THURSDAY | FRIDAY | SATURDAY | SUNDAY |
|---|---|---|---|
| 1 cup oatmeal topped with 1 tablespoon almonds, with 1 cup nonfat milk, 1 cup blueberries | Microwave Quiche in a Mug | 2 slices whole-wheat toast with 2 tablespoons peanut butter, 1 banana, 1 hardboiled egg | Peaches and Greens Smoothie |
| ½ cup canned pineapple, ½ cup low-fat cottage cheese | 1 low-fat string cheese, ½ cup grape tomatoes | 1 apple, 1 cup low-fat Greek yogurt (flavored or plain) | 1 low-fat string cheese, ½ cup grape tomatoes |
| Leftover Easy Roast Salmon with Roasted Asparagus | Leftover Mustard-Crusted Pork Tenderloin in a wrap with Greek Yogurt Mayo | Leftover Orange-Beef Stir-Fry | Leftover Mustard-Crusted Pork Tenderloin in a salad with Cranberry Sauce |
| Banana-Cashew Cream Mousse | 1 apple, ¼ cup almonds | Banana-Cashew Cream Mousse | 1 banana, ¼ cup almonds |
| Mustard-Crusted Pork Tenderloin plus side salad | Orange-Beef Stir-Fry | Leftover Mustard-Crusted Pork Tenderloin in a wrap with Greek Yogurt Mayo | Roasted sliced turkey, sautéed carrots and onions, side salad |

# MICROWAVE QUICHE IN A MUG

**VEGETARIAN**
**30-MINUTE**
**BUDGET-SAVER**

**PREP** 2 minutes
**COOK** 3 minutes

½ cup chopped frozen spinach, thawed and drained (or ½ cup packed fresh spinach)

1 large egg

⅓ cup low-fat milk

1 teaspoon olive oil

1 pinch black pepper

½ slice whole grain bread, torn into small pieces

This recipe also appears in chapter 5, p. 62.

*serves 1* **Busy mornings require nutritious dishes that are quick to prepare. This quiche takes only 5 minutes to make. The best part is that it includes 1 serving of vegetables and is rich in high-quality protein to keep you feeling full.**

1. If using fresh spinach, place it in a mug with 2 table-spoons of water. Cover with a paper towel and microwave for 1 minute. Remove from microwave and drain the water from the spinach before adding it back to the mug. If using frozen spinach, make sure it is completely thawed and drained.

2. Crack the egg into the mug with the spinach and add the milk, olive oil, and pepper. Whisk until thoroughly mixed.

3. Add bread and stir in gently, but do not whisk.

4. Place mug in microwave and cook on high for 1 minute until egg is cooked, and quiche is slightly puffed.

5. Enjoy immediately.

**SUBSTITUTION TIP** You can replace the spinach with 4 halved cherry tomatoes and add them in step two. You could also replace the olive oil with 1 teaspoon of butter. Vary the seasonings to your personal preferences and use your favorite herbs and spices.

---

**Per Serving** Total Calories: 216; Total Fat 11g; Saturated Fat: 3g; Cholesterol: 191mg; Sodium: 268mg; Potassium: 352mg; Total Carbohydrate: 18g; Fiber: 4g; Sugars: 5g; Protein: 14g

# PEACHES AND GREENS SMOOTHIE

**VEGETARIAN**
**30-MINUTE**
**BUDGET-SAVER**

**PREP** 5 minutes

2 cups fresh spinach
(or ⅓ cup frozen)

1 cup frozen peaches
(or fresh, pitted)

1 cup ice

½ cup nonfat or low-fat milk

½ cup plain nonfat
Greek yogurt

½ teaspoon vanilla extract

*Optional:* no-calorie
sweetener of choice

This recipe
also appears
in chapter 5,
p. 66.

*serves 1* **Starting your day with a smoothie is a
quick way to enjoy a nutritious breakfast without
cooking a thing. Creamy and sweet, this meal in a
glass is high in blood-pressure-lowering calcium,
magnesium, and potassium.**

1. Add all of the ingredients to a blender and process
   until smooth.

2. Enjoy immediately.

**INGREDIENT TIP** When making smoothies, frozen ingredients like
spinach and peaches will result in a thicker smoothie. You can always
thin it by adding less ice or more liquid. Alternatively, using fresh
spinach and fresh peaches will result in a thinner smoothie, so adjust
the liquid and ice according to your personal preferences.

**Per Serving** Total Calories: 191; Total Fat: 0g; Saturated
Fat: 0g; Cholesterol: 7mg; Sodium: 157mg; Potassium: 984mg;
Total Carbohydrate: 30g; Fiber: 3g; Sugars: 23g; Protein: 18g

# SOUTHWEST TOFU SCRAMBLE

**VEGAN**
**30-MINUTE**
**ONE POT**

**PREP** 10 minutes
**COOK** 15 minutes

½ tablespoon olive oil

½ red onion, chopped

2 cups chopped spinach

8 ounces firm tofu, drained well

1 teaspoon ground cumin

½ teaspoon garlic powder

*Optional for serving:* sliced avocado, sliced tomatoes

This recipe also appears in chapter 6, p. 74.

*serves 1* **This savory, Southwest-inspired tofu scramble is packed with filling protein and—thanks to the spinach and onions—is high in fiber, calcium, magnesium, and potassium. Soy is considered a complete protein, which means it has all of the amino acids your body needs.**

1. Heat the olive oil in a medium skillet over medium heat. Add the onion and cook until softened, about 5 minutes.

2. Add the spinach and cover to steam for 2 minutes.

3. Using a spatula, move the veggies to one side of the pan. Crumble the tofu into the open area in the pan, breaking it up with a fork. Add the garlic and cumin to the crumbled tofu and mix well. Sauté for 5 to 7 minutes until the tofu is slightly browned.

4. Serve immediately with whole-grain bread, fruit, or beans. Top with sliced avocado and tomato, if using.

**INGREDIENT TIP** If you want your tofu to look and taste like scrambled eggs, add 1 teaspoon of ground turmeric. Hailing from the ginger family, turmeric is deep orange-yellow in color and is a common ingredient in Indian foods. A rich source of anti-inflammatories, turmeric has numerous health benefits.

**Per Serving** Total Calories: 267; Total Fat: 17g; Saturated Fat: 3g; Cholesterol: 0mg; Sodium: 75mg; Potassium: 685mg; Total Carbohydrate: 13g; Fiber: 5g; Sugars: 2g; Protein: 23g

# BAKED CHICKPEA-AND-ROSEMARY OMELET

**VEGETARIAN**
**30-MINUTE**
**ONE POT**
**BUDGET-SAVER**

**PREP** 10 minutes
**COOK** 15 minutes

½ tablespoon olive oil

4 eggs

¼ cup grated
Parmesan cheese

1 (15-ounce) can chickpeas,
drained and rinsed

2 cups packed baby spinach

1 cup button
mushrooms, chopped

2 sprigs rosemary, leaves
picked (or 2 teaspoons dried
rosemary)

Salt

Freshly ground black pepper

This recipe
also appears
in chapter 6,
p. 87.

*serves 2* **Simple, satisfying, and quick to prepare, this recipe helps you meet your goals for protein, calcium, potassium, and magnesium.**

1. Preheat the oven to 400°F and place a baking tray on the middle shelf.

2. Line an 8-inch springform pan with baking paper and grease generously with olive oil. If you don't have a springform pan, grease an oven-safe skillet (or cast-iron skillet) with olive oil.

3. Lightly whisk together the eggs and Parmesan.

4. Place chickpeas in the prepared pan. Layer the spinach and mushrooms on top of the beans. Pour the egg mixture on top and scatter the rosemary. Season to taste with salt and pepper.

5. Place the pan on the preheated tray and bake until golden and puffy and the center feels firm and springy, about 15 minutes.

6. Remove from oven, slice, and serve immediately.

**SUBSTITUTION TIP** You can vary the beans, vegetables, and cheese in this recipe and come up with your own favorite combinations. Try asparagus, goat cheese, and white beans for a delicious variation.

**Per Serving** Total Calories: 418; Total Fat: 19g; Saturated Fat: 6g; Cholesterol: 382mg; Sodium: 595mg; Potassium: 273mg; Total Carbohydrate: 33g; Fiber: 12g; Sugars: 2g; Protein: 30g

# EASY ROAST SALMON WITH ROASTED ASPARAGUS

**30-MINUTE**
**ONE POT**

**PREP** 5 minutes
**COOK** 15 minutes

2 (5-ounce) salmon fillets with skin

2 teaspoons olive oil, plus extra for drizzling

Salt

Freshly ground black pepper

1 bunch asparagus, trimmed

1 teaspoon dried chives

1 teaspoon dried tarragon

Fresh lemon wedges for serving

This recipe also appears in chapter 7, p. 99.

*serves 2* **Salmon is an excellent source of heart-healthy omega-3 fatty acids—for optimum health, recommendations are to include at least 2 servings of salmon, or another fatty fish, each week. This recipe is easy and fancy—a perfect dish for any night of the week.**

1. Preheat the oven to 425°F.

2. Rub salmon all over with 1 teaspoon of olive oil per fillet. Season with salt and pepper.

3. Place asparagus spears on a foil-lined baking sheet and lay the salmon fillets skin-side down on top. Put pan in upper-third of oven and roast until fish is just cooked through, about 12 minutes. Roasting time will vary depending on the thickness of your salmon. Salmon should flake easily with a fork when it's ready and an instant-read thermometer should register 145°F.

4. When cooked, remove from oven, cut fillets in half cross-wise, then lift flesh from skin with a metal spatula and transfer to a plate. Discard skin, then drizzle salmon with oil, sprinkle with herbs, and serve with lemon wedges and roasted asparagus spears.

**BUDGET-SAVER TIP** There is a wide range of price, color, and taste among the six species of salmon we commonly eat, so as with any fish, buy the best salmon you can find and afford. Pink and chum are smaller fish and are good budget choices.

**Per Serving** Total Calories: 353; Total Fat: 22g; Saturated Fat: 4g; Cholesterol: 88mg; Sodium: 90mg; Potassium: 304mg; Total Carbohydrate: 5g; Fiber: 2g; Sugars: 0g; Protein: 34g

# LEMON-PARSLEY BAKED FLOUNDER AND BRUSSELS SPROUTS

**30-MINUTE**

**PREP** 10 minutes
**COOK** 15 minutes

14 Brussels sprouts

2 tablespoons olive oil, divided

3 tablespoons fresh lemon juice

1 tablespoon minced fresh garlic

¼ teaspoon dried dill

2 (6-ounce) flounder fillets

Salt

Freshly ground black pepper

This recipe also appears in chapter 7, p. 102.

*serves 2* **Flounder and other white fish are very low in calories and fat and provide an excellent source of filling protein. And since DASH recommends increasing your intake of vegetables, this recipe makes use of oven time to roast a tray of potassium-rich Brussels sprouts.**

1. Preheat the oven to 400°F. Rinse the Brussels sprouts and pat them dry. Cut the stem end off, cut in half, and place them on a foil-lined baking pan. Drizzle with 1 tablespoon olive oil and toss to coat.

2. Meanwhile in a small bowl, stir together 1 tablespoon olive oil, lemon juice, garlic, and dill.

3. Rinse flounder fillets and pat dry, season lightly with salt and pepper. Place in baking dish and evenly drizzle oil-and-herb mixture over flounder fillets.

4. Bake for 10 to 11 minutes, or until the fish flakes easily when tested with a fork. The Brussels sprouts should be lightly browned and also pierce easily with a fork.

5. Divide the flounder and Brussels sprouts between serving plates.

**INGREDIENT TIP** Roasting vegetables is easy to do and intensifies flavors. For best results, use a shallow pan and don't overcrowd it. Season them with olive oil and your favorite herbs.

**Per Serving** Total Calories: 319; Total Fat: 17g; Saturated Fat: 2g; Cholesterol: 98mg; Sodium: 529mg; Potassium: 538mg; Total Carbohydrate: 13g; Fiber: 5g; Sugars: 3g; Protein: 33g

# MUSTARD-CRUSTED PORK TENDERLOIN

**30-MINUTE
ONE POT**

**PREP** 15 minutes
**COOK** 15 minutes

3 tablespoons Dijon mustard

3 tablespoons honey

1 teaspoon dried rosemary

1 tablespoon olive oil

1 pound pork tenderloin

Salt

Freshly ground black pepper

*This recipe also appears in chapter 8, p. 110.*

*serves 4* **Technically a type of red meat, certain cuts of pork are very lean and low in fat. Pork tenderloin is one of the most tender cuts of pork and is easy to cook. This recipe uses a mustard coating for a juicy result. Serve this dish with a side of steamed vegetables and fresh green salad.**

1. Preheat the oven to 425°F with the rack set in the middle. In a small bowl, combine the Dijon mustard, honey, and rosemary. Stir to combine, set aside.

2. Preheat an oven-safe skillet over high heat and add olive oil. While it is heating up, pat pork loin dry with a paper towel and season lightly with salt and pepper on all sides. When the skillet is hot, sear the pork loin on all sides until golden brown, about 3 minutes per side. Remove from the heat and spread honey-mustard mixture evenly to coat the pork loin.

3. Place the skillet in the oven and cook the pork for 15 minutes, or until an instant-read thermometer registers 145°F.

4. Remove from the oven and allow to rest for 3 minutes. Slice the pork into ½-inch slices and serve.

**INGREDIENT TIP** Pork cooking-temperature guidelines have been revised in recent years because today's pork is more lean and safe. For best results, target an internal pork cooking temperature between 145°F and 160°F. Measure the temperature at the thickest part of the cut. Remember to allow the pork to rest for 3 minutes before serving.

**Per Serving** Total Calories: 220; Total Fat: 9g; Saturated Fat: 3g; Cholesterol: 45mg; Sodium: 307mg; Potassium: 11mg; Total Carbohydrate: 14g; Fiber: 0g; Sugars: 13g; Protein: 19g

# ORANGE-BEEF STIR-FRY

**30-MINUTE
ONE POT**

**PREP** 10 minutes
**COOK** 10 minutes

1 tablespoon cornstarch

¼ cup cold water

¼ cup orange juice

1 tablespoon reduced-sodium soy sauce

½ pound boneless beef sirloin steak, cut into thin strips

2 teaspoons olive oil, divided

3 cups frozen stir-fry vegetable blend

1 garlic clove, minced

This recipe also appears in chapter 8, p. 115.

*serves 2* **This orange-beef stir-fry may just become one of your favorite go-to recipes when you need to put a healthy dinner on the table fast. Full of flavor and color, this 2-serving recipe will satisfy that craving for takeout in a healthy, DASH-friendly way. This dish is high in lean protein and vitamin- and mineral-rich vegetables, with a kick of spice from the red pepper flakes.**

1. In a small bowl, combine the cornstarch, cold water, orange juice, and soy sauce until smooth. Set aside.

2. In a large skillet or wok, stir-fry beef in 1 teaspoon oil for 3 to 4 minutes or until no longer pink. Remove with a slotted spoon and keep warm.

3. Stir-fry the vegetable blend and garlic in the remaining oil for 3 minutes. Stir cornstarch mixture and add to the pan. Bring to a boil; cook and stir for 2 minutes or until thickened. Add beef and heat through.

**BUDGET-SAVER TIP** Buy the amount of beef your budget allows. You can reduce the beef by half and add in 1 cup of frozen protein-rich edamame. This would also help you to practice taking the focus off meat in a meal and making it more plant-based.

**Per Serving** Total Calories: 268; Total Fat: 10g; Saturated Fat: 3g; Cholesterol: 65mg; Sodium: 376mg; Potassium: 65mg; Total Carbohydrate: 8g; Fiber: 3g; Sugars: 8g; Protein: 26g

# CARROT-CAKE SMOOTHIE

**VEGETARIAN**
**30-MINUTE**
**BUDGET-SAVER**

**PREP** 5 minutes

1 frozen banana, peeled and diced

1 cup carrots, diced (peeled if preferred)

1 cup nonfat or low-fat milk

½ cup nonfat or low-fat vanilla Greek yogurt

½ cup ice

¼ cup diced pineapple, frozen

½ teaspoon ground cinnamon

Pinch nutmeg

*Optional toppings:* chopped walnuts, grated carrots

This recipe also appears in chapter 9, p. 131.

*serves 2* **Enjoy a classic dessert favorite in the form of a healthier smoothie. This nutritious carrot-cake smoothie is made with antioxidant- and potassium-rich carrots, calcium, and protein-rich Greek yogurt, and has all of the taste of traditional carrot cake with the addition of pineapple, walnuts, and carrot-cake spices.**

1. Add all of the ingredients to a blender and process until smooth and creamy.

2. Serve immediately with optional toppings as desired.

**INGREDIENT TIP** You could also use plain Greek yogurt or plain regular yogurt and add your own sweetener to this recipe. Good choices are 1 to 2 teaspoons of pure maple syrup or honey. You could also opt for a no-calorie sweetener like stevia.

---

**Per Serving** Total Calories: 180; Total Fat: 1g; Saturated Fat: 0g; Cholesterol: 5mg; Sodium: 114mg; Potassium: 682mg; Total Carbohydrate: 36g; Fiber: 4g; Sugars: 25g; Protein: 10g

# BANANA-CASHEW CREAM MOUSSE

**VEGETARIAN**

**PREP** 55 minutes, plus 2 to 3 hours for soaking cashews

½ cup cashews, presoaked

1 tablespoon honey

1 teaspoon vanilla extract

1 large banana, sliced (reserve 4 slices for garnish)

1 cup plain nonfat Greek yogurt

This recipe also appears in chapter 9, p. 135.

*serves 2* **This quick Banana-Cashew Cream Mousse recipe makes and unbelievably satisfying and heart-healthy snack or dessert. Perfectly suited to the DASH eating plan, each serving contains ample amounts of calcium, magnesium, potassium, healthy fats, and protein. It can help you to meet your goals for several food groups including dairy, nuts, and protein. Light and fluffy with a creamy texture, you can even eat this for breakfast.**

1. Place the cashews in a small bowl and cover with 1 cup of water. Soak at room temperature for 2 to 3 hours. Drain, rinse, and set aside.

2. Place honey, vanilla extract, cashews, and bananas in a blender or food processor. Blend until smooth.

3. Place mixture in a medium bowl. Fold in yogurt, mix well. Cover.

4. Chill in refrigerator, covered, for at least 45 minutes.

5. Portion mousse into 2 serving bowls. Garnish each with 2 banana slices.

**INGREDIENT TIP** Soaking nuts is thought to remove their enzyme inhibitors and reduce their phytic acid content, making them easier to digest and their nutrients more easily absorbed. Soaking may also remove potential irritants such as mold and pesticides.

**Per Serving** Total Calories: 329; Total Fat: 14g; Saturated Fat: 3g; Cholesterol: 8mg; Sodium: 64mg; Potassium: 507mg; Total Carbohydrate: 37g; Fiber: 3g; Sugars: 24g; Protein: 17g

# CRANBERRY SAUCE

**VEGAN**
**ONE POT**
**BUDGET-SAVER**

**PREP** 5 minutes
**COOK** 10 minutes, plus
30 minutes cooling time

½ cup sugar

½ cup water

1 (12-ounce) package fresh
or frozen cranberries

½ teaspoon ground cinnamon

*Optional:* 2 tablespoons
100% orange juice

This recipe
also appears
in chapter 10,
p. 145.

*makes 2¼ cups* **Cranberries have an amazing array of phytonutrients that offer cardio-vascular and immune support, protection against urinary-tract infections, and anti-inflammatory benefits. One of the most nutrient-rich berries out there, cranberries are inexpensive and are available year round, fresh or frozen. This simple recipe uses just a couple of ingredients. Serve this delicious sauce as a side to cooked fish or meat.**

1. Combine all the ingredients in a medium saucepan. Bring to a boil over medium-high heat, then reduce to a simmer. Cook, stirring occasionally, until berries start to pop. Press berries against side of pan with a wooden spoon and continue to cook, until berries are completely broken down and achieve a jam-like consistency, about 10 minutes total.

2. Remove from heat and allow to cool for about 30 minutes. Stir in water in 1 tablespoon increments to adjust to desired consistency.

3. Serve immediately or store in the refrigerator for 10 to 14 days. You can also freeze the sauce and, for best results, aim to use it within 1 to 2 months.

**BUDGET-SAVER TIP** Buy several bags of cranberries when they are in season and on sale. Store them in the freezer without opening or washing. When ready to use, simply wash and drain.

**Per ¼ Cup Serving** Total Calories: 113; Total Fat: 0g; Saturated Fat: 0g; Cholesterol: 0mg; Sodium: 0mg; Potassium: 1mg; Total Carbohydrate: 29g; Fiber: 3g; Sugars: 26g; Protein: 0g

# GREEK YOGURT MAYONNAISE

**VEGETARIAN**
**30-MINUTE**
**BUDGET-SAVER**

**PREP** 2 minutes

6 ounces nonfat or low-fat plain Greek yogurt

1 teaspoon apple cider vinegar

¼ teaspoon yellow mustard

¼ teaspoon hot sauce

¼ teaspoon pepper

¼ teaspoon paprika

¼ teaspoon salt

This recipe also appears in chapter 10, p. 146.

*serves 12* **Mayonnaise is not known as a healthy condiment, even though it is a staple in many homes. You can make a much healthier spread that's high in DASH-recommended nutrients in just a few minutes. Greek yogurt has a similar thick consistency and works as a great base for a homemade version. Greek yogurt is also high in calcium and is packed with protein (keeping you feeling full) and probiotics that aid in digestion. Adjust the spices to suit your tastes.**

Mix all the ingredients together and blend well. Adjust seasonings to suit taste.

**INGREDIENT TIP** Greek yogurt is a staple you might consider keeping on hand when following the DASH diet. Try it as an alternative for heavy cream, add a pinch of salt and use in place of sour cream, add spices and a bit of milk for a creamy salad dressing, or simply enjoy plain as a snack.

**Per 2-Tablespoon Serving** Total Calories: 8; Total Fat: 0g; Saturated Fat: 0g; Cholesterol: 0mg; Sodium: 65mg; Potassium: 2mg; Total Carbohydrate: 1g; Fiber: 0g; Sugars: 1g; Protein: 1g

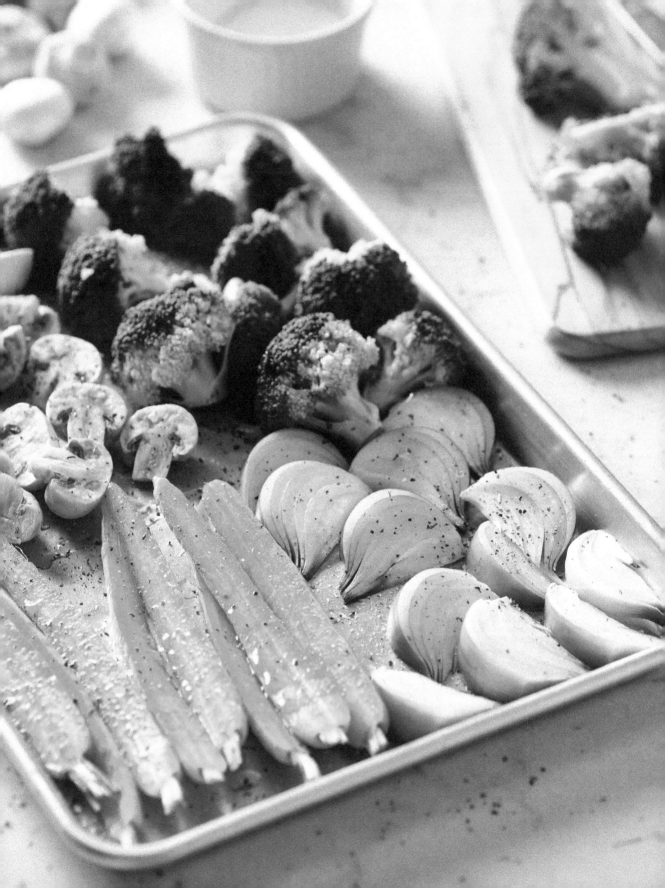

# *four*
# Week Two Meal Plan & Recipes

**This chapter features the second week** of the meal plan, which includes another seven days of menus that conform to the DASH diet. The meal plans are written for a single person, so if you are cooking for more than yourself, you will need to double the shopping lists and recipes. Twelve recipes from this book were used to create each meal plan. The shopping list includes the items needed to make the 12 recipes from the meal plan. Lunches from this week will be leftovers from the previous nights' dinner recipes, so none will be included. A very basic pantry list is also provided and these basic staples were used in the Week 1 Meal Plan to limit the number of items you need to purchase to get started on following the DASH diet.

The recipes needed to prepare the meals in the meal plans are included in this chapter. The recipes will be grouped together by meal and appear in the meal plan's order of appearance. Not all meals will require recipes and instead suggestions will be made for what to eat so that you can use these menus as a basis for your own healthy meal planning. If a suggested meal or snack option doesn't appeal to you, simply make a DASH-friendly substitute using the recipes in this book. Remember that on some days you may eat a few more or less recommended servings of a particular food group. That's okay, as long as the average for the week is close to the recommendations. The exception is sodium. Try to stay within the daily limit for sodium (1,500 mg) as much as possible.

# WEEK TWO SHOPPING LIST

This list outlines everything you need to make all the recipes for the week for one person to follow the plan.

## PANTRY LIST

- ☐ Almonds, unsalted
- ☐ Cooking spray, nonstick
- ☐ Garlic
- ☐ Olive oil
- ☐ Onions
- ☐ Peanut butter, unsalted
- ☐ Pepper
- ☐ Rolled oats
- ☐ Salt

## REFRIGERATED STAPLES

- ☐ Fruit, fresh
- ☐ Milk, nonfat or low-fat
- ☐ Salad greens

## FRESH PRODUCE

- ☐ Apples (2)
- ☐ Bananas (3)
- ☐ Orange (1)
- ☐ Lemon (1)
- ☐ Spinach (2 cups)
- ☐ Tomatoes, plum (4)
- ☐ Tomatoes, slicing (2 large)
- ☐ Zucchini (1)
- ☐ Garlic (6 cloves)
- ☐ Onions, red (2 large)
- ☐ Onions, yellow (2 large)
- ☐ Mushrooms (2 cups)
- ☐ Vegetables, fresh, of your choosing (2 cups)
- ☐ Peppers, bell (6)

*Optional for toppings*
- ☐ Avocado (1)
- ☐ Tomato (1)
- ☐ Onion (1)

## OILS, VINEGARS & CONDIMENTS

- ☐ Olive oil
- ☐ Lime juice
- ☐ Lemon juice
- ☐ Vinegar, balsamic
- ☐ Vinegar, white

## DRY GOODS

- ☐ Rice, brown (½ cup)
- ☐ Sugar, brown (3 tablespoons)
- ☐ Sugar (1 cup)
- ☐ Oats, rolled (1 cup)
- ☐ Pasta, whole-wheat, angel hair (4 ounces)
- ☐ Walnuts (4 tablespoons)

## CANNED & BOTTLED GOODS

- ☐ Chickpeas (1 [15-ounce] can)
- ☐ Beans, black (1 [15-ounce] can)
- ☐ Beans, red (1 [15-ounce] can)
- ☐ Beans, white (1 [5-ounce] can)
- ☐ Chipotle peppers, in adobo sauce (1 [7-ounce] can)

## DAIRY & EGGS

- ☐ Milk, nonfat or low-fat (2 cups)
- ☐ Cheese, Parmesan, grated (2 tablespoons)
- ☐ Yogurt, Greek, nonfat or low-fat, plain (2½ cups)
- ☐ String cheese, low-fat (1 pack)

## MEAT & SEAFOOD, PLUS MEAT ALTERNATIVES

- ☐ Steaks (2 [4-ounce] filets)
- ☐ Pork chops, boneless (4)
- ☐ Shrimp (4 ounces)
- ☐ Chicken, skinless and boneless (2 [4-ounce] breasts)

## FREEZER

- ☐ Strawberries (2 cups)
- ☐ Spinach (10 ounces)

## SEASONINGS & FLAVORINGS

- ☐ Basil, dried
- ☐ Cinnamon
- ☐ Cumin
- ☐ Oregano, dried
- ☐ Red pepper, crushed
- ☐ Thyme, dried

# WEEK TWO MENU

| | MONDAY | TUESDAY | WEDNESDAY |
|---|---|---|---|
| *breakfast* | Overnight Oats with Bananas and Walnuts | 2 hardboiled eggs, 2 slices turkey bacon with ½ cup grape tomatoes, 1 apple, 2 slices whole-wheat toast | Strawberry Yogurt Smoothie |
| *snack* | 1 apple, 1 cup low-fat Greek yogurt (flavored or plain) | 1 banana, 1 cup low-fat Greek yogurt (flavored or plain) | 1 low-fat string cheese, ½ cup baby carrots |
| *lunch* | Leftover White Beans with Spinach and Pan-Roasted Tomatoes | Leftover Balsamic-Roasted Chicken Breasts with Spiced Pepper Relish | Leftover Red Beans and Rice with Fresh Vegetable Salsa |
| *snack* | Roasted Chickpeas and baby carrots | ½ cup grape tomatoes, ¼ cup almonds | Roasted Chickpeas and baby carrots |
| *dinner* | Balsamic-Roasted Chicken Breasts with side salad | Red Beans and Rice with Fresh Vegetable Salsa and side salad | Shrimp Pasta Primavera with side salad |

| THURSDAY | FRIDAY | SATURDAY | SUNDAY |
|---|---|---|---|
| 1 cup low-fat Greek yogurt (flavored or plain) with ½ cup blueberries and 2 tablespoons almonds, 1 slice whole-wheat toast with 1 slice cheese and tomato slices | Overnight Oats with Bananas and Walnuts | 2 slices whole-wheat toast with 2 table-spoons peanut butter, 1 banana, 1 hardboiled egg | Strawberry Yogurt Smoothie |
| ½ cup canned pineapple, ½ cup low-fat cottage cheese | 1 low-fat string cheese, ½ cup grape tomatoes | 1 apple, 1 cup low-fat Greek yogurt (flavored or plain) | 1 low-fat string cheese, ½ cup grape tomatoes |
| Leftover Shrimp Pasta Primavera | Leftover Apple-Cinnamon Baked Pork Chops | Leftover Grilled Steak, Onions, and Mushrooms | Leftover Apple-Cinnamon Baked Pork Chops |
| Chunky Black-Bean Dip with Bell Pepper Strips | 1 cup low-fat Greek yogurt (flavored or plain), ¼ cup almonds | Chunky Black-Bean Dip with Bell Pepper Strips | 1 hardboiled egg, ½ cup baby carrots |
| Apple-Cinnamon Baked Pork Chops with side salad | Grilled Steak, Onions, and Mushrooms | Leftover Apple-Cinnamon Baked Pork Chops | White Beans with Spinach and Pan-Roasted Tomatoes |

# OVERNIGHT OATS WITH BANANAS AND WALNUTS

**VEGETARIAN**
**BUDGET-SAVER**

**PREP** 5 minutes, plus 8 hours at rest

½ cup rolled oats

½ cup low-fat milk

1 ripe banana, mashed

2 tablespoons chopped walnuts

¼ teaspoon ground cinnamon

*Optional:* no-calorie sweetener of choice

*This recipe also appears in chapter 5, p. 64.*

*serves 1* **Overnight oats are a no-cook, no-bake, super-nutritious breakfast—prepared in minutes after soaking the mixture overnight in the refrigerator. No lingering by the stove, waiting for oats to simmer and thicken. Simply add a few basic ingredients to a jar or bowl. Overnight, the oats absorb the milk and flavors, forming a delicious and creamy grab-and-go breakfast. With whole grains, fruits, and nuts, overnight oats are DASH-certified!**

1. To a Mason jar or container of choice, add the oats, mashed banana, walnuts, and cinnamon. Pour in the milk and gently stir until combined.

2. Place in the refrigerator overnight or for at least 8 hours.

3. When ready to serve, top with additional milk if desired.

**BUDGET-SAVER TIP** You can replace the walnuts with chopped unsalted peanuts or mix in ½ tablespoon of unsalted natural peanut butter. All nuts are nutritious and high in heart-healthy fats, so purchase the type of nut or nut butter that fits within your budget.

**Per Serving** Total Calories: 405; Total Fat: 15g; Saturated Fat: 2g; Cholesterol: 8mg; Sodium: 62mg; Potassium: 492mg; Total Carbohydrate: 62g; Fiber: 8g; Sugars: 21g; Protein: 13g

# STRAWBERRY YOGURT SMOOTHIE

**VEGETARIAN**
**BUDGET-SAVER**

**PREP** 5 minutes

1 cup plain nonfat or low-fat Greek yogurt

1 cup frozen strawberries

1 cup ice

½ cup nonfat or low-fat milk

½ orange, peeled

½ frozen banana

*This recipe also appears in chapter 5, p. 67.*

*serves 1* Sweet, juicy strawberries are not only delicious, they are low in calories, a good source of fiber, and loaded with plant chemicals called *phytochemicals* that contain protective disease-preventive compounds. With their blood-pressure-lowering abilities, this little berry adds just the right amount of sweetness to this nutritious smoothie.

1. Add all of the ingredients to a blender and process until smooth.

2. Enjoy immediately.

**INGREDIENT TIP** Frozen bananas are used in many smoothie recipes as they add a sweet flavor and a creamy, thick consistency. Whenever you have overripe bananas, peel and slice them, and freeze them in freezer bags so you have them on hand for smoothie making.

**Per Serving** Total Calories: 305; Total Fat: 1g; Saturated Fat: 0g; Cholesterol: 13mg; Sodium: 170mg; Potassium: 1,284mg; Total Carbohydrate: 52g; Fiber: 6g; Sugars: 37g; Protein: 29g

# RED BEANS AND RICE

**VEGAN**
**BUDGET-SAVER**

**PREP** 5 minutes
**COOK** 45 minutes

½ cup dry brown rice

1 cup water, plus ¼ cup

1 (15-ounce) can red beans, drained and rinsed

1 tablespoon ground cumin

Juice of 1 lime

4 handfuls fresh spinach

*Optional toppings:* avocado, chopped tomatoes, Greek yogurt, onions

*This recipe also appears in chapter 6, p. 77.*

*serves 2* **This recipe is inexpensive, quick, easy, and helps boost your intake of beans and whole grains, which meets the DASH-diet recommendations. The base is simple yet the possibilities for toppings and add-ins are endless.**

1. Combine rice and water in a pot and bring to a boil. Cover and reduce heat to a low simmer. Cook for 30 to 40 minutes or according to package directions.

2. Meanwhile, add the beans, ¼ cup of water, cumin, and lime juice to a medium skillet. Bring to a boil. Reduce to a simmer and let cook until most of the liquid is absorbed, 5 to 7 minutes.

3. Once the liquid is mostly gone, remove from the heat and add the spinach. Cover and let spinach wilt slightly, 2 to 3 minutes. Mix in with the beans.

4. Serve beans with rice. Add toppings, if using.

**INGREDIENT TIP** Keep your freezer stocked with an assortment of frozen vegetables including spinach, broccoli, cauliflower, summer squash, and peppers. Add your favorites to boost the fiber and vitamins and minerals in this recipe.

**Per Serving** Total Calories: 232; Total Fat: 2g; Saturated Fat: 0g; Cholesterol: 0mg; Sodium: 210mg; Potassium: 228mg; Total Carbohydrate: 41g; Fiber: 12g; Sugars: 1g; Protein: 13g

# WHITE BEANS WITH SPINACH AND PAN-ROASTED TOMATOES

**VEGAN**
**30-MINUTE**
**ONE POT**
**BUDGET-SAVER**

**PREP** 15 minutes
**COOK** 10 minutes

1 tablespoon olive oil

4 small plum tomatoes, halved lengthwise

10 ounces frozen spinach, defrosted and squeezed of excess water

2 garlic cloves, thinly sliced

2 tablespoons water

¼ teaspoon freshly ground black pepper

1 (15-ounce) can white beans, drained and rinsed

Juice of 1 lemon

This recipe also appears in chapter 6, p. 81.

*serves 2* White beans—like cannellini, kidney, and navy—are packed with plant protein, fiber, iron, B vitamins, and potassium. They are also a budget-friendly staple that can be used in endless ways. In this recipe, tomatoes (which are rich in vitamin C) are pan-roasted and combined with beans and magnesium-rich spinach in a delicious one-pot meal with all of the nutrients you need to lower your blood pressure.

1. Heat the oil in a large skillet over medium-high heat. Add the tomatoes, cut-side down, and cook, shaking the pan occasionally, until browned and starting to soften, 3 to 5 minutes; turn and cook for 1 minute more. Transfer to a plate.

2. Reduce heat to medium and add the spinach, garlic, water, and pepper to the skillet. Cook, tossing, until the spinach is heated through, 2 to 3 minutes.

3. Return the tomatoes to the skillet, add the white beans and lemon juice, and toss until heated through, 1 to 2 minutes.

**INGREDIENT TIP** Consider purchasing a jar of minced garlic for use in recipes. Jarred garlic has a long shelf life, cuts down on food waste, and reduces preparation time.

**Per Serving** Total Calories: 293; Total Fat: 9g; Saturated Fat: 1g; Cholesterol: 0mg; Sodium: 267mg; Potassium: 648mg; Total Carbohydrate: 43g; Fiber: 16g; Sugars: 1g; Protein: 15g

# BALSAMIC-ROASTED CHICKEN BREASTS

**ONE POT**

**PREP** 35 minutes
**COOK** 40 minutes

¼ cup balsamic vinegar

1 tablespoon olive oil

2 teaspoons dried oregano

2 garlic cloves, minced

2 (4-ounce) boneless, skinless, chicken-breast halves

½ teaspoon freshly ground black pepper

⅛ teaspoon salt

Cooking spray

*This recipe also appears in chapter 7, p. 97.*

*serves 2* **Baked balsamic chicken is wholesome, delicious, and very easy to make. Marinating the chicken breasts makes the meat extra tender and juicy. You can customize the recipe to use whatever herbs you have on hand. A good source of lean protein, chicken breast is very low in calories and is a good source of B vitamins, which are important for heart health.**

1. In a small bowl, add the vinegar, oil, oregano, garlic, salt, and pepper. Mix to combine.

2. Put the chicken in a resealable plastic bag. Pour the vinegar mixture in the bag with the chicken, seal the bag, and coat the chicken to marinate. Refrigerate for 30 minutes.

3. Preheat the oven to 400°F. Spray a small baking dish with cooking spray.

4. Put the chicken in prepared baking dish and pour the marinade over the chicken. Cover and bake for 35 to 40 minutes, or until an instant-read thermometer registers 165°F.

5. Let sit for 5 minutes, then serve with your favorite vegetables.

**BUDGET-SAVER TIP** Quick-cooking grain medleys are a healthy choice that make it easy and budget friendly to increase your consumption of whole grains. Several name brands offer brown-rice and whole-grain medleys that can be prepared in just 10 minutes.

**Per Serving** Total Calories: 226; Total Fat: 11g; Saturated Fat: 3g; Cholesterol: 65mg; Sodium: 129mg; Potassium: 44mg; Total Carbohydrate: 6g; Fiber: 1g; Sugars: 0g; Protein: 25g

# SHRIMP PASTA PRIMAVERA

**30-MINUTE**
**ONE POT**

**PREP** 5 minutes
**COOK** 15 minutes

2 tablespoons olive oil

1 tablespoon garlic, minced

2 cups assorted fresh
vegetables, chopped coarsely
(zucchini, broccoli, asparagus,
whatever you prefer)

4 ounces frozen shrimp,
cooked, peeled, and deveined

Salt

Freshly ground black pepper

Juice of ½ lemon

4 ounces whole-wheat
angel-hair pasta, cooked per
package instructions

2 tablespoons grated
Parmesan cheese

*This recipe
also appears
in chapter 7,
p. 100.*

*serves 2* This low-calorie, well-seasoned,
flavorful pasta dish comes together in just minutes, and is easy on the budget. Shrimp are low
in calories and are protein-rich—and while they
do contain cholesterol, dietary cholesterol has a
minimal impact on blood cholesterol. *Primavera*
in Italian means "spring," as in "a mixture of fresh
spring vegetables," so feel free to use your favorites
to customize this recipe.

1. Heat the oil in a large nonstick skillet over medium heat.
   Add the garlic and sauté for 1 minute.

2. Add vegetables and sauté until crisp tender, 3 to 4 minutes.

3. Add the shrimp and sauté until just heated through. Season
   lightly with salt and pepper and squeeze lemon juice over
   the shrimp and vegetables. Continue to cook for about
   2 minutes until the juices have been reduced by about half.
   Remove from heat.

4. Toss shrimp and vegetables with pasta. Serve topped with
   Parmesan cheese.

**BUDGET-SAVER TIP** You can cut down on cost by replacing the
fresh vegetables with a 16-ounce bag of frozen mixed vegetables.
Read the ingredients list and make sure that there is no added salt
or seasonings.

**Per Serving** Total Calories: 439; Total Fat: 17g; Saturated
Fat: 3g; Cholesterol: 105mg; Sodium: 286mg; Potassium: 481mg;
Total Carbohydrate: 50g; Fiber: 8g; Sugars: 5g; Protein: 23g

# APPLE-CINNAMON BAKED PORK CHOPS

**ONE POT**

**PREP** 10 minutes
**COOK** 40 minutes

2 apples, peeled, cored, and sliced

1 teaspoon ground cinnamon, divided

4 boneless pork chops (½-inch thick)

Salt

Freshly ground black pepper

¾ cup water

3 tablespoons brown sugar

1 tablespoon olive oil

This recipe also appears in chapter 8, p. 111.

*serves 4* **This satisfying sweet and savory dish pairs simple ingredients and pantry staples to create a delicious flavor combination. Pork chops are a budget-friendly protein and apples are available year round, making this an inexpensive yet healthy dinner that can help you meet your fruit and protein servings for the day. Serve this dish with a side of steamed green beans.**

1. Preheat the oven to 375°F. Layer apples in bottom of casserole dish. Sprinkle with ½ teaspoon of cinnamon.

2. Trim fat from pork chops. Lay on top of the apple slices. Sprinkle with a dash of salt and pepper.

3. In a small bowl, combine ¾ cup of water, brown sugar, and remaining cinnamon. Pour the mixture over the chops. Drizzle chops with 1 tablespoon of olive oil.

4. Bake uncovered in preheated oven for 30 to 45 minutes or until an instant-read thermometer registers between 145°F and 160°F. Allow to rest for 3 minutes before serving.

**INGREDIENT TIP** To enhance the taste of this dish, substitute 100 percent apple juice or apple cider in place of the water. Be certain to read the ingredients list and choose a variety without added sugar.

**Per Serving** Total Calories: 244; Total Fat: 10g; Saturated Fat: 3g; Cholesterol: 45mg; Sodium: 254mg; Potassium: 124mg; Total Carbohydrate: 22g; Fiber: 4g; Sugars: 19g; Protein: 21g

# GRILLED STEAK, ONIONS, AND MUSHROOMS

**30-MINUTE**

**PREP** 5 minutes
**COOK** 25 minutes

1 tablespoon olive oil, plus enough for grill rack

2 (4-ounce) filet steaks (1½-inches thick)

Salt

Freshly ground black pepper

2 cups sliced mushrooms

1 cup sliced red onion

This recipe also appears in chapter 8, p. 117.

*serves 2* **This protein-packed dish is low in sodium and fat. It includes 3 servings of vegetables in each portion. Aim to limit your consumption of red meat to an occasional treat, and when you do choose red meat, fill half of your plate with vegetables, which is easy to do with this recipe.**

1. Prepare a grill for high heat. Apply olive oil to the grill rack.

2. Sprinkle steaks lightly with salt and pepper.

3. Place steaks on grill with direct high heat and sear for 1 to 2 minutes per side. Reduce heat to medium and cook for 18 to 23 minutes, or until done according to your preference, turning once during cooking. Transfer steaks to a plate and cover with foil; let rest for 5 minutes before serving.

4. In a medium sauté pan, heat the oil over medium-high heat on the grill. Add mushrooms and onions and sauté for 5 to 6 minutes until tender.

5. Serve the steak with the mushrooms and onions and a fresh green salad.

**INGREDIENT TIP** You can also "grill" indoors by heating olive oil in a medium skillet over high heat, adding the steak and searing for about 3 minutes per side, until the steak is deep brown and crisp. Allow the meat to rest for 5 to 10 minutes before serving.

**Per Serving** Total Calories: 345; Total Fat: 23g; Saturated Fat: 7g; Cholesterol: 75mg; Sodium: 63mg; Potassium: 220mg; Total Carbohydrate: 8g; Fiber: 3g; Sugars: 1g; Protein: 26g

# CHUNKY BLACK-BEAN DIP

**VEGETARIAN**
**30-MINUTE**
**BUDGET-SAVER**

**YIELD** 2 cups
**PREP** 5 minutes

1 (15-ounce) can black
beans, drained, with liquid
reserved

½ (7-ounce) can chipotle
peppers in adobo sauce

¼ cup nonfat or low-fat
plain Greek yogurt

Freshly ground black pepper

This recipe
also appears
in chapter 9,
p. 127.

*serves 6–8* **This black-bean dip makes a
healthy snack and can help you increase your
intake of beans and dairy, two DASH-recommended
foods. Made with just three main ingredients, this
dip is full of flavor and goes great paired with raw
vegetables, mixed into hot grains, or used as a
sandwich spread.**

1. Combine beans, peppers, and yogurt in a food processor
   or blender and process until smooth. Add some of the bean
   liquid, 1 tablespoon at a time, for a thinner consistency.

2. Season to taste with black pepper.

3. Serve.

**INGREDIENT TIP** Chipotles are small peppers that have been dried
by a smoking process that gives them a dark color and a distinct
smoky flavor. You can find this canned ingredient in the Latin aisle of
grocery stores and big-box chains. As an alternative, you could use
1 teaspoon dry chipotle chili powder.

**Per ⅓-Cup Serving** Total Calories: 70; Total Fat: 1g; Saturated
Fat: 0g; Cholesterol: 0mg; Sodium: 159mg; Potassium: 21mg; Total
Carbohydrate: 11g; Fiber: 4g; Sugars: 0g; Protein: 5g

# ROASTED CHICKPEAS

**VEGAN**
**ONE POT**
**BUDGET-SAVER**

**PREP** 5 minutes
**COOK** 30 minutes

1 (15-ounce can) chickpeas, drained and rinsed

½ teaspoon olive oil

2 teaspoons of your favorite herbs or spice blend

¼ teaspoon salt

This recipe also appears in chapter 9, p. 130.

*serves 2* **Following a healthy diet doesn't mean you have to give up crunchy, tasty snacks. Remember, you always want to think of how you can *add* nutrients to your diet. So with that principle in mind, this simple roasted-chickpeas recipe uses a handful of pantry ingredients to create a delicious, nutritious, crunchy, positively addictive snack that you can feel good about eating.**

1. Preheat the oven to 400°F.

2. Drain and rinse the chickpeas. Spread a layer of paper towels on a rimmed baking sheet and spread the chickpeas on top. Blot the top with more paper towels until the chickpeas are relatively dry.

3. Place the dried chickpeas in a medium bowl. Drizzle in the olive oil and toss gently with a large spoon. Sprinkle on the herbs and salt and toss again.

4. Spread chickpeas on the baking sheet in a single layer.

5. Bake for 30 to 40 minutes, stirring halfway through, until golden brown and crunchy.

6. Serve.

**INGREDIENT TIP** If you like everything bagels, try mixing together 1 teaspoon each: sesame seeds, poppy seeds, dried minced onion, and dried minced garlic—use this mixture as the seasoning in this recipe to make everything-roasted chickpeas.

**Per Serving** Total Calories: 175; Total Fat: 3g; Saturated Fat: 0g; Cholesterol: 0mg; Sodium: 474mg; Potassium: 0mg; Total Carbohydrate: 29g; Fiber: 11g; Sugars: 0g; Protein: 11g

# FRESH VEGETABLE SALSA

**VEGETARIAN**
**30-MINUTE**
**ONE POT**

**PREP** 10 minutes

2 cups cored and diced bell peppers

2 cups diced tomatoes

1 cup diced zucchini

½ cup chopped red onion

¼ cup freshly squeezed lime juice

2 garlic cloves, minced

1 teaspoon freshly ground black pepper

¼ teaspoon salt

This recipe also appears in chapter 10, p. 147.

*makes 6 cups* **Store-bought salsa is surprisingly high in sodium and, while the DASH diet doesn't restrict sodium, too much of this mineral can contribute to high blood pressure. Making your own fresh salsa is easy, and this recipe uses a mix of vegetables high in potassium and magnesium, keeping added salt in check. Adapt this recipe to your personal preferences for heat and types of vegetables.**

1. Wash the vegetables and prepare as directed.

2. In a large bowl, combine all the ingredients. Toss gently to mix.

3. Cover and refrigerate for at least 30 minutes to allow the flavors to blend.

**SUBSTITUTION TIP** If you prefer hotter salsa, add ½ to 1 tablespoon of finely chopped, seeded jalapeño peppers. You could also make this a bean salsa by adding ½ cup of black or pinto beans.

**Per ¼-Cup Serving** Total Calories: 10; Total Fat: 0g; Saturated Fat: 0g; Cholesterol: 0mg; Sodium: 26mg; Potassium: 81mg; Total Carbohydrate: 2g; Fiber: 1g; Sugars: 1g; Protein: 0g

# SPICED PEPPER RELISH

**VEGAN**
**ONE POT**
**BUDGET-SAVER**

**PREP** 5 minutes
**COOK** 35 minutes

4 red bell peppers, cored and shredded

2 large onions, shredded

1 cup sugar

1 cup white wine vinegar

½ cup water

½ teaspoon salt

1 teaspoon crushed red pepper

*This recipe also appears in chapter 10, p. 149.*

*makes 5 cups* Adding vegetable relish to sandwiches or salads or spooning it over beans, are great ways to sneak more vegetables into your diet, without even noticing it. Homemade relish is very easy to make, is inexpensive, and can be stored in the refrigerator for up to a month. This relish recipe is similar to traditional sweet-pickle relish but with a peppery kick.

1. Combine all the ingredients in a large saucepan and bring to a boil. Reduce heat, and simmer, uncovered, for 35 minutes or until thick, stirring frequently.

2. Cool, pour into airtight containers, and store in the refrigerator for up to 1 month.

**INGREDIENT TIP** Relish can be mixed into Greek yogurt to make a dip, puréed into a salad dressing, served on burgers, and mixed into ground meats. Get creative in the ways you boost your daily intake of vegetables.

**Per 2-Tablespoon Serving** Total Calories: 28; Total Fat: 0g; Saturated Fat: 0g; Cholesterol: 0mg; Sodium: 30mg; Potassium: 52mg; Total Carbohydrate: 7g; Fiber: 0g; Sugars: 5g; Protein: 0g

# PART TWO

# Recipes for DASH Living

All of the recipes in this book are designed to yield one to four servings, use five main ingredients or fewer, are low in sodium and saturated fat, and are high in vitamins, minerals, and fiber. The use of specialty items is avoided. The ingredients used are all budget friendly and readily available at grocery stores and big-box chains. The ingredients have also been selected for their high content of nutrients—including calcium, magnesium, and potassium—shown to reduce blood pressure.

Recipe labels will help you quickly learn more about the attributes of the recipes. Labels include:

**VEGETARIAN AND VEGAN**
Vegetarian recipes may contain eggs or dairy. Vegan recipes do not contain any animal products.

**30-MINUTE**
The recipes can be prepared and served in 30 minutes or less.

**ONE POT AND SHEET PAN**
The recipes require only one pot or one sheet pan to cook.

**BUDGET-SAVER**
A budget-saver recipe costs less than $5 per serving and usually contains frozen, canned, and dried ingredients.

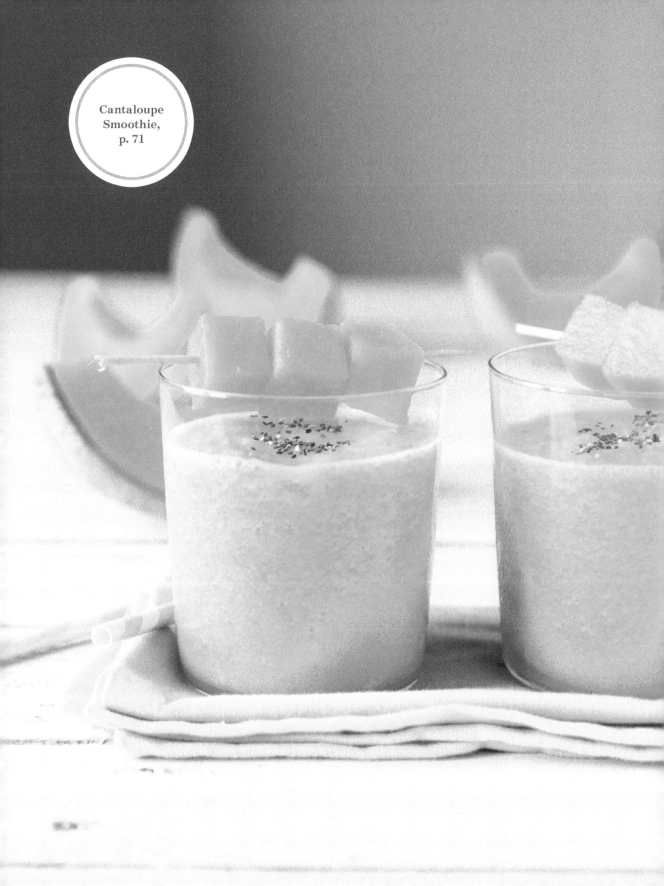

Cantaloupe
Smoothie,
p. 71

# Breakfasts & Smoothies

*five*

Microwave Quiche
in a Mug **62**

Avocado and Egg Toast **63**

Overnight Oats with
Bananas and Walnuts **64**

Steel-Cut Oats with
Blueberries and Almonds **65**

Peaches and Greens
Smoothie **66**

Strawberry Yogurt
Smoothie **67**

Peanut Butter and
Banana Smoothie **68**

Make-Ahead Fruit and
Yogurt Parfait **69**

Blueberry-Oatmeal
Muffin in a Mug **70**

Cantaloupe Smoothie **71**

# MICROWAVE QUICHE IN A MUG

**VEGETARIAN**
**30-MINUTE**
**BUDGET-SAVER**

**PREP** 2 minutes
**COOK** 3 minutes

½ cup chopped frozen spinach, thawed and drained (or ½ cup packed fresh spinach)

1 large egg

⅓ cup low-fat milk

1 teaspoon olive oil

Freshly ground black pepper

½ slice whole-grain bread, torn into small pieces

*serves 1* Busy mornings require nutritious dishes that are quick to prepare. And this quiche takes only 5 minutes to make. The best part is that it includes 1 serving of vegetables and is rich in high-quality protein to keep you feeling full.

1. If using fresh spinach, place it in a mug with 2 tablespoons of water. Cover with a paper towel and microwave for 1 minute. Remove from microwave and drain the water from the spinach before adding it back to the mug. If using frozen spinach, make sure it is completely thawed and drained.

2. Crack the egg into the mug with the spinach and add the milk, olive oil, and pepper. Whisk until thoroughly mixed.

3. Add bread and stir in gently, but do not whisk.

4. Place mug in the microwave and cook on high for 1 minute until egg is cooked, and quiche is slightly puffed.

5. Enjoy immediately.

**SUBSTITUTION TIP** You can replace the spinach with 4 halved cherry tomatoes and add them in step 2. You could also replace the olive oil with 1 teaspoon of butter. Vary the seasonings to your personal preferences and use your favorite herbs and spices.

**Per Serving** Total Calories: 216; Total Fat 11g; Saturated Fat: 3g; Cholesterol: 191mg; Sodium: 268mg; Potassium: 352mg; Total Carbohydrate: 18g; Fiber: 4g; Sugars: 5g; Protein: 14g

# AVOCADO AND EGG TOAST

VEGETARIAN
30-MINUTE
BUDGET-SAVER

**PREP** 5 minutes
**COOK** 5 minutes

2 eggs

2 slices whole-grain bread

1 small avocado

1 teaspoon freshly squeezed lime juice

Freshly ground black pepper

*serves 1* With more potassium per serving than a banana, avocados make an excellent choice on the DASH eating plan. The fruit is incredibly nutritious, boasting high amounts of cholesterol-lowering fiber, heart-healthy monounsaturated fats, and 20 different vitamins and minerals. Simple and quick, this recipe includes a serving of protein, fruit, and whole grains with a flavor and texture combination that's delicious.

1. Toast bread and cook eggs to personal preference.

2. Peel and mash avocado with the lime juice and pepper.

3. Spread avocado evenly on each slice of toast, then top each with a fried egg.

4. Serve immediately.

**INGREDIENT TIP** When it comes to choosing avocados, skin color is not always the best indicator for ripeness. Ultimately, an avocado's ripeness is determined by how it yields to gentle pressure, and ripe avocados that yield to this should be eaten within 1 to 2 days.

**Per Serving** Total Calories: 612; Total Fat: 38g; Saturated Fat: 7g; Cholesterol: 372mg; Sodium: 535mg; Potassium: 1,015mg; Total Carbohydrate: 50g; Fiber: 18g; Sugars: 7g; Protein: 24g

# OVERNIGHT OATS WITH BANANAS AND WALNUTS

**VEGETARIAN
BUDGET-SAVER**

**PREP** 5 minutes, plus
8 hours at rest

½ cup rolled oats

½ cup nonfat or low-fat milk

1 ripe banana, mashed

2 tablespoons
chopped walnuts

¼ teaspoon ground cinnamon

*Optional:* no-calorie
sweetener of choice

*serves 1* Overnight oats are a no-cook, no-bake, super-nutritious breakfast—prepared in minutes after soaking the mixture overnight in the refrigerator. No lingering by the stove, waiting for oats to simmer and thicken. Simply add a few basic ingredients to a jar or bowl. Overnight the oats absorb the milk and flavors, forming a delicious and creamy grab-and-go breakfast. With whole grains, fruits, and nuts, overnight oats are DASH-certified!

1. To a Mason jar or container of choice, add the oats, mashed banana, walnuts, and cinnamon. Pour in the milk and gently stir until combined.

2. Place in the refrigerator overnight or for at least 8 hours.

3. When ready to serve, top with additional milk if desired.

**BUDGET-SAVER TIP** You can replace the walnuts with chopped unsalted peanuts or mix in ½ tablespoon unsalted natural peanut butter. All nuts are nutritious and high in heart-healthy fats so purchase the type of nut or nut butter that fits within your budget.

---

**Per Serving** Total Calories: 405; Total Fat: 15g; Saturated Fat: 2g; Cholesterol: 8mg; Sodium: 62mg; Potassium: 492mg; Total Carbohydrate: 62g; Fiber: 8g; Sugars: 21g; Protein: 13g

# STEEL-CUT OATS WITH BLUEBERRIES AND ALMONDS

**VEGETARIAN**
**30-MINUTE**
**BUDGET-SAVER**

**PREP** 10 minutes
**COOK** 17 minutes

1 cup nonfat or low-fat milk

1 cup water

1 teaspoon ground cinnamon

1 cup steel-cut oats

1 cup blueberries

½ cup sliced almonds

*serves 4* **Whole grains are vital to a healthy DASH lifestyle and steel-cut oats offer a chewier, nuttier alternative to rolled oats. Processed differently from rolled oats, steel-cut oats are made from oat kernels that have been cut into thick pieces so they take longer to digest. An excellent source of slow-burning energy and cholesterol-lowering fiber, this filling breakfast can contribute to lower blood pressure.**

1. In a medium saucepan over medium heat, whisk together milk, water, and cinnamon.

2. When the mixture starts to come to a boil, add steel-cut oats and bring to a boil.

3. Reduce heat to low and simmer for 15 minutes.

4. About 2 minutes before the end of cooking time, add in blueberries and almonds and stir well.

5. Serve immediately.

**BUDGET-SAVER TIP** Purchase frozen berries to keep costs in check. Any type of berry will work in this recipe—and all berries are nutritious and heart healthy, as they are high in antioxidants, vitamins, minerals, and fiber.

**Per Serving** Total Calories: 268; Total Fat: 10g; Saturated Fat: 1g; Cholesterol: 1mg; Sodium: 28mg; Potassium: 241mg; Total Carbohydrate: 39g; Fiber: 7g; Sugars: 7g; Protein: 11g

# PEACHES AND GREENS SMOOTHIE

**VEGETARIAN**
**30-MINUTE**
**BUDGET-SAVER**

**PREP** 5 minutes

2 cups fresh spinach
(or ⅓ cup frozen)

1 cup frozen peaches
(or fresh, pitted)

1 cup ice

½ cup nonfat or low-fat milk

½ cup plain nonfat or
low-fat Greek yogurt

½ teaspoon vanilla extract

*Optional:* no-calorie
sweetener of choice

*serves 1* **Starting your day with a smoothie is a quick way to enjoy a nutritious breakfast, without cooking a thing. Creamy and sweet, this meal in a glass is high in blood-pressure-lowering calcium, magnesium, and potassium.**

1. Add all of the ingredients to a blender and process until smooth.

2. Enjoy immediately.

**INGREDIENT TIP** When making smoothies, frozen ingredients like frozen spinach and peaches will result in a thicker smoothie. You can always thin it by adding less ice or more liquid. Alternatively, using fresh spinach and fresh peaches will result in a thinner smoothie, so adjust the liquid and ice according to your personal preferences.

**Per Serving** Total Calories: 191; Total Fat: 0g; Saturated Fat: 0g; Cholesterol: 7mg; Sodium: 157mg; Potassium: 984mg; Total Carbohydrate: 30g; Fiber: 3g; Sugars: 23g; Protein: 18g

# STRAWBERRY YOGURT SMOOTHIE

**VEGETARIAN**
**BUDGET-SAVER**

**PREP** 5 minutes

1 cup plain nonfat or low-fat Greek yogurt

1 cup frozen strawberries

1 cup ice

½ cup nonfat or low-fat milk

½ orange, peeled

½ frozen banana

*serves 1* **Sweet, juicy strawberries are not only delicious, they are low in calories, a good source of fiber, and loaded with plant chemicals called *phytochemicals* that contain protective disease-preventive compounds. With their blood-pressure-lowering abilities, this little berry adds just the right amount of sweetness to this nutritious smoothie.**

1. Add all of the ingredients to a blender and process until smooth.

2. Enjoy immediately.

**INGREDIENT TIP** Frozen bananas are used in many smoothie recipes as they add a sweet flavor and a creamy, thick consistency. Whenever you have overripe bananas, peel and slice them, and freeze them in freezer bags so you have them on hand for smoothie making.

**Per Serving** Total Calories: 305; Total Fat: 1g; Saturated Fat: 0g; Cholesterol: 13mg; Sodium: 170mg; Potassium: 1,284mg; Total Carbohydrate: 52g; Fiber: 6g; Sugars: 37g; Protein: 29g

# PEANUT BUTTER AND BANANA SMOOTHIE

**VEGETARIAN**
**30-MINUTE**
**BUDGET-SAVER**

**PREP** 5 minutes

1 cup nonfat or low-fat milk

1 cup ice

¼ cup plain nonfat or low-fat Greek yogurt

1 frozen banana, sliced

1 tablespoon peanut butter

*serves 1* **The DASH diet encourages the consumption of nuts several times a week for their abilities to promote heart health and aid in weight management. Peanuts are high in heart-healthy monounsaturated fats, and are good sources of vitamin E, niacin, folate, and protein. As creamy and delicious as it is nutritious, this smoothie is also full of calcium and potassium, essential nutrients that promote healthy blood pressure.**

1. Add all of the ingredients to a blender and process until smooth.

2. Enjoy immediately.

**INGREDIENT TIP** Experiment with the amount of liquid and ice you use in smoothies until you find your desired level of thickness. You can add 1 to 2 tablespoons of rolled oats to any of the smoothie recipes for added fiber and a small portion of whole grains. Oats also add a nice touch of sweetness and make smoothies thicker.

---

**Per Serving** Total Calories: 313; Total Fat: 9g; Saturated Fat: 2g; Cholesterol: 8mg; Sodium: 136mg; Potassium: 1,037mg; Total Carbohydrate: 45g; Fiber: 5g; Sugars: 30g; Protein: 19g

# MAKE-AHEAD FRUIT AND YOGURT PARFAIT

VEGETARIAN
30-MINUTE
BUDGET-SAVER

**PREP** 10 minutes

¾ cup plain nonfat or low-fat Greek yogurt

⅓ cup rolled oats

2 tablespoons nonfat or low-fat milk

1 apple, skin left on, washed, cored, and diced

2 tablespoons chopped walnuts

*serves 1* This easy, make-ahead breakfast is packed with plenty of protein and heart-healthy fats to give you energy all morning long. Apples contain a type of fiber called pectin, which can help reduce bad LDL cholesterol. With a serving each of dairy, fruit, whole grains, and healthy fats, make several of these parfaits at once for grab-and-go breakfasts all week long.

1. In a bowl, combine yogurt, oats, and milk. Stir to combine.

2. Layer half of the yogurt mixture in a wide-mouth Mason jar or container. Add half of the apple and 1 tablespoon of the walnuts, then layer in remaining yogurt mixture and top with remaining apple and nuts.

3. Cover and refrigerate overnight and up to 5 days.

**SUBSTITUTION TIP** Some other combinations you may want to try include: blackberries and crushed graham crackers; raspberries, sliced almonds, and lemon zest; pineapple, mango, and pistachios.

**Per Serving** Total Calories: 355; Total Fat: 12g; Saturated Fat: 1g; Cholesterol: 8mg; Sodium: 99mg; Potassium: 614mg; Total Carbohydrate: 43g; Fiber: 6g; Sugars: 21g; Protein: 24g

# BLUEBERRY-OATMEAL MUFFIN IN A MUG

VEGETARIAN
30-MINUTE
BUDGET-SAVER

**PREP** 1 minute
**COOK** 1 minute

½ cup rolled oats

1 egg

2 tablespoons nonfat or low-fat milk

⅓ cup blueberries

Cooking spray

*Optional:* no-calorie sweetener of choice

*serves 1* **Swap your high-calorie bakery muffin for this filling and nutritious oatmeal muffin—which you can make in minutes. Bursting with antioxidant-rich blueberries, packed with fiber-rich oats, and loaded with filling protein, this single-serve muffin tastes more like dessert than breakfast. The recipe also makes a nutritious snack or dessert.**

1. Spray a large mug or small ramekin with cooking spray.

2. Add the oats, egg, and milk, and stir to combine. Gently fold in the blueberries.

3. Place in the microwave and cook on high for 1 minute, being careful to watch as it could overflow. If the muffin does not look firm, place back in for 30 seconds at a time.

4. Once ready, flip mug upside down onto a plate, slice, and enjoy.

**INGREDIENT TIP** You can also make this in the oven: Preheat the oven to 350°F, place the mug or dish on the center rack, and bake for 20 minutes or until the muffin is set.

**Per Serving** Total Calories: 259; Total Fat: 8g; Saturated Fat: 2g; Cholesterol: 187mg; Sodium: 87mg; Potassium: 159mg; Total Carbohydrate: 36g; Fiber: 5g; Sugars: 8g; Protein: 13g

# CANTALOUPE SMOOTHIE

**VEGETARIAN**
**30-MINUTE**
**BUDGET-SAVER**

**PREP** 5 minutes

½ cup nonfat or low-fat milk

1 frozen banana, sliced

1 (5.3-ounce) carton vanilla nonfat Greek yogurt

½ cup ice

1 teaspoon honey

2½ cups (1-inch) cubed and peeled frozen cantaloupe

*serves 2* **When following the DASH diet, cantaloupe is one of the fruits you will want to enjoy more often. A very good source of the mineral potassium, 1 cup has over 12 percent of your recommended daily intake. This nutritious fruit is also an excellent source of the antioxidant vitamin C and a good source of the mineral magnesium, B vitamins, and fiber. Creamy and delicious, each serving also provides one of your dairy and protein servings for the day, keeping you feeling full.**

1. Place the milk, banana, yogurt, ice, and honey in a blender—process until smooth.

2. Add the cantaloupe pieces and process until smooth.

3. Serve immediately.

**BUDGET-SAVER TIP** An economical and healthy way to add protein to smoothies, soups, and other recipes is to add a couple of tablespoons of nonfat dry milk powder to the ingredients. Nonfat dry milk powder has all of the nutritional attributes of fluid nonfat milk, only is in powdered form. If you don't drink much milk and are afraid of spoilage, consider adding some dry milk to your pantry staples.

**Per Serving** Total Calories: 214; Total Fat: 1g; Saturated Fat: 0g; Cholesterol: 4mg; Sodium: 67mg; Potassium: 994mg; Total Carbohydrate: 46g; Fiber: 3g; Sugars: 38g; Protein: 11g

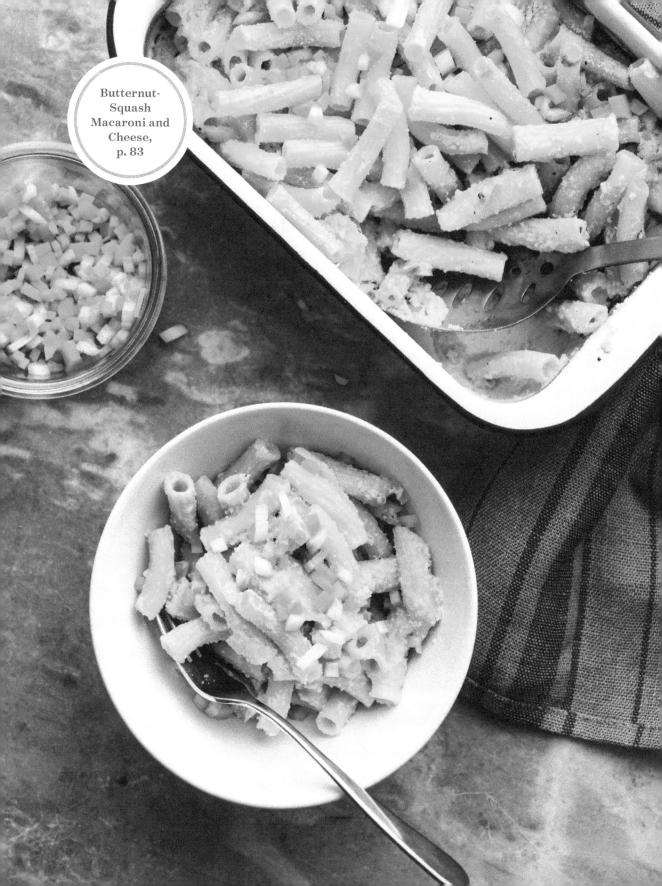

Butternut-
Squash
Macaroni and
Cheese,
p. 83

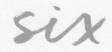

# Vegetarian & Vegan Mains

Southwest Tofu
Scramble **74**

Black-Bean and
Vegetable Burrito **75**

Baked Eggs in Avocado **76**

Red Beans and Rice **77**

Hearty Lentil Soup **78**

Black-Bean Soup **79**

Loaded Baked Sweet
Potatoes **80**

White Beans with
Spinach and Pan-Roasted
Tomatoes **81**

Black-Eyed Peas and
Greens Power Salad **82**

Butternut-Squash
Macaroni and Cheese **83**

Pasta with Tomatoes
and Peas **84**

Healthy Vegetable
Fried Rice **85**

Portobello-Mushroom
Cheeseburgers **86**

Baked Chickpea-and-
Rosemary Omelet **87**

Chilled Cucumber-and-
Avocado Soup with Dill **88**

Easy Chickpea Veggie
Burgers **89**

# SOUTHWEST TOFU SCRAMBLE

VEGAN
30-MINUTE
ONE POT

**PREP** 10 minutes
**COOK** 15 minutes

½ tablespoon olive oil

½ red onion, chopped

2 cups chopped spinach

8 ounces firm tofu, drained well

1 teaspoon ground cumin

½ teaspoon garlic powder

*Optional for serving:* sliced avocado or sliced tomatoes

*serves 1* This savory, Southwest-inspired tofu scramble is packed with filling protein and—thanks to the spinach and onions—is high in fiber, calcium, magnesium, and potassium. Soy is considered a complete protein, which means it has all of the amino acids your body needs.

1. Heat the olive oil in a medium skillet over medium heat. Add the onion and cook until softened, about 5 minutes.

2. Add the spinach and cover to steam for 2 minutes.

3. Using a spatula, move the veggies to one side of the pan. Crumble the tofu into the open area in the pan, breaking it up with a fork. Add the cumin and garlic to the crumbled tofu and mix well. Sauté for 5 to 7 minutes until the tofu is slightly browned.

4. Serve immediately with whole-grain bread, fruit, or beans. Top with optional sliced avocado and tomato, if using.

**INGREDIENT TIP** If you want your tofu to look and taste like scrambled eggs, add 1 teaspoon of ground turmeric. Hailing from the ginger family, turmeric is deep orange-yellow in color and is a common ingredient in Indian foods. A rich source of anti-inflammatories, turmeric has numerous health benefits.

**Per Serving** Total Calories: 267; Total Fat: 17g; Saturated Fat: 3g; Cholesterol: 0mg; Sodium: 75mg; Potassium: 685mg; Total Carbohydrate: 13g; Fiber: 5g; Sugars: 2g; Protein: 23g

# BLACK-BEAN AND VEGETABLE BURRITO

**VEGAN**
**30-MINUTE**
**ONE POT**

**PREP** 10 minutes
**COOK** 15 minutes

½ tablespoon olive oil

2 red or green bell peppers, cored and chopped

1 zucchini or summer squash, diced

½ teaspoon chili powder

1 teaspoon cumin

Freshly ground black pepper

2 (15-ounce) cans black beans, drained and rinsed

1 cup cherry tomatoes, halved

4 (8-inch) whole-wheat tortillas

*Optional for serving:* spinach, sliced avocado, chopped scallions, or hot sauce

*serves 4* Burritos—literally meaning "little donkeys"—are a staple of Southwestern cuisine. They can be made with a few basic pantry staples and customized to suit your personal preferences. Healthy, quick, filling, and delicious, once you master the basic recipe this can be a go-to meal for when you need a DASH-friendly dish fast.

1. Heat the oil in a large sauté pan over medium heat. Add the bell peppers and sauté until crisp tender, about 4 minutes.

2. Add the zucchini, chili powder, cumin, and black pepper to taste, and continue to sauté until the vegetables are tender, about 5 minutes.

3. Add the black beans and cherry tomatoes and cook until the tomatoes soften, the beans are heated through, and most of the moisture has evaporated, about 5 minutes.

4. Divide between 4 burritos and serve topped with optional ingredients as desired.

5. Enjoy immediately.

**INGREDIENT TIP** The possibilities are endless when it comes to burritos and the types of beans and vegetables you choose. Try chickpeas with red peppers, edamame with shredded purple cabbage, or pinto beans with mushrooms.

**Per Serving** Total Calories: 311; Total Fat: 6g; Saturated Fat: 1g; Cholesterol: 0mg; Sodium: 499mg; Potassium: 400mg; Total Carbohydrate: 52g; Fiber: 21g; Sugars: 1g; Protein: 19g

# BAKED EGGS IN AVOCADO

VEGETARIAN
30-MINUTE
BUDGET-SAVER

**PREP** 10 minutes
**COOK** 15 minutes

2 avocados

Juice of 2 limes

Freshly ground black pepper

4 eggs

2 (8-inch) whole-wheat or corn tortillas, warmed

*Optional for serving:* halved cherry tomatoes and chopped cilantro

*serves 2* This filling and delicious recipe requires just a few ingredients and nearly no prep time. Avocados are a good source of cholesterol-lowering fiber and heart-healthy fats, and eggs are a budget-friendly source of high-quality protein, vitamin D, and many different vitamins and minerals. Served with a whole-wheat tortilla, this meal will keep you feeling full and energized.

1. Adjust oven rack to the middle position and preheat the oven to 450°F.

2. Cut each avocado in half and remove the pit. Using a spoon, scrape out the center of each halved avocado so that it is large enough to accommodate an egg (about 1½ tablespoons). Squeeze lime juice over the avocados and season with black pepper to taste, then place on a baking sheet. Break an egg into the center of each avocado. Don't worry if some of the white spills out, as long as the yolk is intact.

3. Bake in the oven until whites are set and yolk is runny, about 10 to 15 minutes.

4. Remove from oven and garnish with optional cilantro and cherry tomatoes and serve with warm tortillas.

**INGREDIENT TIP** To keep costs in check and minimize the need to purchase fresh herbs, stock your pantry with a variety of dried herbs such as chives and cilantro. You might also consider buying a bottle of lime juice instead of using fresh limes to cut down on potential waste.

---

**Per Serving** Total Calories: 534; Total Fat: 39g; Saturated Fat: 8g; Cholesterol: 372mg; Sodium: 462mg; Potassium: 1,095mg; Total Carbohydrate: 30g; Fiber: 20g; Sugars: 3g; Protein: 23g

# RED BEANS AND RICE

VEGAN
BUDGET-SAVER

PREP 5 minutes
COOK 45 minutes

½ cup dry brown rice

1 cup water, plus ¼ cup

1 (15-ounce) can red beans, drained and rinsed

1 tablespoon ground cumin

Juice of 1 lime

4 handfuls fresh spinach

*Optional toppings:* avocado, chopped tomatoes, Greek yogurt, onions

*serves 2* **This recipe is inexpensive, quick, easy, and helps boost your intake of beans and whole grains, which meets the DASH-diet recommendations. The base is simple yet the possibilities for toppings and add-ins are endless.**

1. Combine rice and water in a pot and bring to a boil. Cover and reduce heat to a low simmer. Cook for 30 to 40 minutes or according to package directions.

2. Meanwhile, add the beans, ¼ cup of water, cumin, and lime juice to a medium skillet. Bring to a boil. Reduce to a simmer and let cook until most of the liquid is absorbed, 5 to 7 minutes.

3. Once the liquid is mostly gone, remove from the heat and add the spinach. Cover and let spinach wilt slightly, 2 to 3 minutes. Mix in with the beans.

4. Serve beans with rice. Add toppings, if using.

INGREDIENT TIP Keep your freezer stocked with an assortment of frozen vegetables including spinach, broccoli, cauliflower, summer squash, and peppers. Add your favorites to boost the fiber and vitamins and minerals in this recipe.

**Per Serving** Total Calories: 232; Total Fat: 2g; Saturated Fat: 0g; Cholesterol: 0mg; Sodium: 210mg; Potassium: 228mg; Total Carbohydrate: 41g; Fiber: 12g; Sugars: 1g; Protein: 13g

# HEARTY LENTIL SOUP

VEGAN
ONE POT
BUDGET-SAVER

**PREP** 10 minutes
**COOK** 30 minutes

1 tablespoon olive oil

2 carrots, peeled and chopped

2 celery stalks, diced

1 onion, chopped

1 teaspoon dried thyme

½ teaspoon garlic powder

Freshly ground black pepper

1 (28-ounce) can no-salt diced tomatoes, drained

1 cup dry lentils

5 cups water

Salt

*serves 4* Lentils are small, oval legumes that are about the size of a pencil eraser. Compared to other beans, lentils cook quickly and absorb flavors from other foods and seasonings. A nutritional powerhouse, lentils are high in plant protein and fiber, and are a rich source of magnesium and folate. This hearty and nourishing soup is certain to become a household favorite.

1. Heat the oil in a large Dutch oven or pot over medium heat. Once the oil is simmering, add the carrot, celery, and onion. Cook, stirring often, until the onion has softened and is turning translucent, about 5 minutes. Add the thyme, garlic powder, and black pepper. Cook until fragrant while stirring constantly, about 30 seconds.

2. Pour in the drained diced tomatoes and cook for a few more minutes, stirring often, in order to enhance their flavor.

3. Add the lentils, water, and a pinch of salt. Raise the heat and bring to a boil, then partially cover the pot and reduce heat to maintain a gentle simmer. Cook for 30 minutes, or until lentils are tender but still hold their shape.

4. Ladle into serving bowls and serve with a fresh green salad and whole-grain bread.

**INGREDIENT TIP** While lentils cook very quickly, you can also buy canned lentils, which would reduce the cooking time of this recipe. Canned lentils are also nice to have on hand to add to salads, burritos, pastas, and rice dishes.

**Per Serving** Total Calories: 168; Total Fat: 4g; Saturated Fat: 1g; Cholesterol: 0mg; Sodium: 130mg; Potassium: 239mg; Total Carbohydrate: 35g; Fiber: 14g; Sugars: 8g; Protein: 10g

# BLACK-BEAN SOUP

VEGAN
30-MINUTE
ONE POT
BUDGET-SAVER

**PREP** 5 minutes
**COOK** 20 minutes

1 yellow onion

1 tablespoon olive oil

2 (15-ounce) cans black beans, drained and rinsed

1 cup diced fresh tomatoes

5 cups low-sodium vegetable broth

¼ teaspoon freshly ground black pepper

¼ cup chopped fresh cilantro

*serves 4* Soups are an excellent food to include in a weight-loss plan, as long as they are done right. Broth-based soups are filling and are relatively low in calories compared to their serving size. Bean-based soups in particular are great choices due to their high fiber and protein content. This soup comes together quickly with a handful of basic pantry staples.

1. In a large saucepan, cook the onion in the olive oil over medium heat until softened, about 4 to 5 minutes.

2. Add the black beans, tomatoes, vegetable broth, and black pepper. Bring to a boil, then reduce heat and simmer for about 15 minutes.

3. Remove from the heat and working in batches ladle the soup into a blender and process until somewhat smooth. Return the soup to the pot, add the cilantro and heat until warmed through.

4. Serve immediately.

**INGREDIENT TIP** Immersion blenders are small handheld blenders that chop, purée, mince, and blend—these tools are perfect for puréeing soups right in the pot. Typically priced at under $20, immersion blenders have a slim stick design that fits right into mixing bowls and pots.

**Per Serving** Total Calories: 234; Total Fat: 5g; Saturated Fat: 1g; Cholesterol: 0mg; Sodium: 363mg; Potassium: 145mg; Total Carbohydrate: 37g; Fiber: 13g; Sugars: 3g; Protein: 11g

# LOADED BAKED SWEET POTATOES

**VEGETARIAN**
**30-MINUTE**

**PREP** 10 minutes
**COOK** 20 minutes

4 sweet potatoes

½ cup nonfat or low-fat plain Greek yogurt

Freshly ground black pepper

1 teaspoon olive oil

1 red bell pepper, cored and diced

½ red onion, diced

1 teaspoon ground cumin

1 (15-ounce) can chickpeas, drained and rinsed

*serves 4* Sweet potatoes may be one of the best sources of beta-carotene, an antioxidant that can reduce inflammation in the body. And while many people think starchy foods are not good choices, sweet potatoes are rich in fiber and have been shown to improve blood-sugar regulation in people with diabetes. Low in calories and high in potassium, this healthy loaded-sweet-potato recipe takes less than 30 minutes to prepare.

1. Poke holes in the potatoes with a fork and cook on your microwave's potato setting until potatoes are soft and cooked through, about 8 to 10 minutes for 4 potatoes. If you don't have a microwave, bake at 400°F for about 45 minutes.

2. Combine the yogurt and black pepper in a small bowl and mix well.

3. Heat the oil in a medium pot over medium heat. Add bell pepper, onion, cumin, and additional black pepper to taste.

4. Add the chickpeas, stir to combine, and heat through, about 5 minutes.

5. Slice the potatoes lengthwise down the middle and top each half with a portion of the bean mixture followed by 1 to 2 tablespoons of the yogurt.

6. Serve immediately.

**INGREDIENT TIP** Nonfat or low-fat Greek yogurt is used in place of higher-calorie and higher-fat sour cream. The thicker consistency of Greek yogurt makes it a perfect swap for sour cream—plus Greek yogurt contains more protein and calcium.

**Per Serving** Total Calories: 264; Total Fat: 2g; Saturated Fat: 0g; Cholesterol: 1mg; Sodium: 124mg; Potassium: 428mg; Total Carbohydrate: 51g; Fiber: 10g; Sugars: 1g; Protein: 11g

# WHITE BEANS WITH SPINACH AND PAN-ROASTED TOMATOES

**VEGAN**
**30-MINUTE**
**ONE POT**
**BUDGET-SAVER**

**PREP** 15 minutes
**COOK** 10 minutes

1 tablespoon olive oil

4 small plum tomatoes, halved lengthwise

10 ounces frozen spinach, defrosted and squeezed of excess water

2 garlic cloves, thinly sliced

2 tablespoons water

¼ teaspoon freshly ground black pepper

1 (15-ounce) can white beans, drained and rinsed

Juice of 1 lemon

*serves 2* **White beans—like cannellini, kidney, and navy—are packed with plant protein, fiber, iron, B vitamins, and potassium. They are also a budget-friendly staple that can be used in endless ways. In this recipe, tomatoes (which are rich in vitamin C) are pan-roasted and combined with beans and magnesium-rich spinach in a delicious one-pot meal with all of the nutrients you need to lower your blood pressure.**

1. Heat the oil in a large skillet over medium-high heat. Add the tomatoes, cut-side down, and cook, shaking the pan occasionally, until browned and starting to soften, 3 to 5 minutes; turn and cook for 1 minute more. Transfer to a plate.

2. Reduce heat to medium and add the spinach, garlic, water, and pepper to the skillet. Cook, tossing, until the spinach is heated through, 2 to 3 minutes.

3. Return the tomatoes to the skillet, add the white beans and lemon juice, and toss until heated through, 1 to 2 minutes.

**INGREDIENT TIP** Consider purchasing a jar of minced garlic for use in recipes. Jarred garlic has a long shelf life, cuts down on food waste, and reduces preparation time.

**Per Serving** Total Calories: 293; Total Fat: 9g; Saturated Fat: 1g; Cholesterol: 0mg; Sodium: 267mg; Potassium: 648mg; Total Carbohydrate: 43g; Fiber: 16g; Sugars: 1g; Protein: 15g

# BLACK-EYED PEAS AND GREENS POWER SALAD

VEGAN
30-MINUTE
BUDGET-SAVER

PREP  5 minutes
COOK  6 minutes

1 tablespoon olive oil

3 cups purple cabbage, chopped

5 cups baby spinach

1 cup shredded carrots

1 (15-ounce) can black-eyed peas, drained and rinsed

Juice of ½ lemon

Salt

Freshly ground black pepper

*serves 2*  **One of the secrets to weight management is eating foods high in volume yet low in calories. Vegetable-based salads are extremely low in calories yet are high in fiber, vitamins, and minerals. With the addition of a source of protein, they become the perfect meal to fuel you up while keeping calories in check. This power-packed salad meets several of your daily vegetable and protein recommendations on the DASH eating plan, and it tastes delicious, too!**

1. In a medium pan, add the oil and cabbage and sauté for 1 to 2 minutes on medium heat.

2. Next add in your spinach, cover for 3 to 4 minutes on medium heat, until greens are wilted.

3. Remove from the heat and add to a large bowl.

4. Add in the carrots, black-eyed peas, and a splash of lemon juice.

5. Season with salt and pepper, if desired.

6. Toss together and serve.

**INGREDIENT TIP**  If you want to cook black-eyed peas from scratch, first place 2 cups of peas in a pot and cover with water and 1 tablespoon of apple cider vinegar. Let soak for 1 hour or more. Rinse, then refill pot with water, add a dash of salt, and simmer peas for 2 hours over medium heat, until tender. Rinse, drain, and keep in an airtight container until ready to eat.

**Per Serving**  Total Calories: 320; Total Fat: 9g; Saturated Fat: 1g; Cholesterol: 0mg; Sodium: 351mg; Potassium: 544mg; Total Carbohydrate: 49g; Fiber: 18g; Sugars: 10g; Protein: 16g

# BUTTERNUT-SQUASH MACARONI AND CHEESE

**PREP** 10 minutes
**COOK** 20 minutes

1 cup whole-wheat ziti macaroni

2 cups peeled and cubed butternut squash

1 cup nonfat or low-fat milk, divided

Freshly ground black pepper

1 teaspoon Dijon mustard

1 tablespoon olive oil

¼ cup shredded low-fat cheddar cheese

*serves 2* **Did you know that 1 cup of butternut squash has more potassium than a banana, provides over 400 percent of your daily recommended intake of vitamin A (beta-carotene), and contains a healthy dose of vitamins B and C, folate, and fiber? Butternut squash cooks up nice and creamy, reducing the amount of cheese needed in recipes like the classic macaroni-and-cheese dish. A healthy take on a family favorite, this recipe can be prepared in less than 30 minutes.**

1. Cook the pasta al dente.

2. In a medium saucepan, add the butternut squash and ½ cup milk, and place over medium-high heat. Season with black pepper. Bring to a simmer. Reduce heat to low, cover, and cook until fork tender, 8 to 10 minutes.

3. To a blender, add squash and Dijon mustard. Purée until smooth.

4. Meanwhile, place a large sauté pan over medium heat and add olive oil. Add the squash purée and remaining ½ cup of milk. Bring to a simmer and cook until thickened, 5 minutes. Add the cheese and stir to combine.

5. Add the pasta to the sauté pan and stir to combine.

6. Serve immediately.

**INGREDIENT TIP** Cubed and peeled butternut squash can be found in the frozen section or in the produce section of major grocery stores and most big-box chains.

**Per Serving** Total Calories: 373; Total Fat: 10g; Saturated Fat: 2g; Cholesterol: 8mg; Sodium: 193mg; Potassium: 783mg; Total Carbohydrate: 59g; Fiber: 10g; Sugars: 8g; Protein: 14g

# PASTA WITH TOMATOES AND PEAS

VEGAN
30-MINUTE
BUDGET-SAVER

PREP 10 minutes
COOK 15 minutes

½ cup whole-grain pasta
of choice

8 cups water, plus ¼ for
finishing

1 cup frozen peas

1 tablespoon olive oil

1 cup cherry tomatoes, halved

¼ teaspoon freshly ground
black pepper

1 teaspoon dried basil

¼ cup grated Parmesan
cheese (low-sodium)

*serves 2* There is a lot of misinformation concerning the role of pasta in a healthy diet. Whole-grain pasta is a good source of cholesterol-lowering fiber, heart-health-promoting B vitamins, and slow-burning energy. The problem is that most people eat portion sizes that are too large. This fresh and delicious pasta recipe keeps portions in check while making use of vegetables that are high in blood-pressure-lowering nutrients. Serve it warm or cold as a pasta salad.

1. Cook the pasta al dente.

2. Add the water to the same pot you used to cook the pasta, and when it's boiling add the peas. Cook until tender but still firm, about 5 minutes. Drain and set aside.

3. Heat the oil in a large skillet over medium heat. Add the cherry tomatoes, put a lid on the skillet and let the tomatoes soften for about 5 minutes, stirring a few times.

4. Season with black pepper and basil.

5. Toss in the pasta, peas, and ¼ cup of water, stir and remove from the heat.

6. Serve topped with Parmesan.

INGREDIENT TIP If it's been a while since you have shopped for pasta, it may surprise you how many varieties are available in major grocery stores. You can find pasta from big brands made from lentils and chickpeas, and ones with added protein from peas and vegetable-based varieties. These are definitely DASH-friendly choices, so stock your pantry with some new types.

---

**Per Serving** Total Calories: 266; Total Fat: 12g; Saturated Fat: 4g; Cholesterol: 10mg; Sodium: 320mg; Potassium: 313mg; Total Carbohydrate: 30g; Fiber: 6g; Sugars: 5g; Protein: 13g

# HEALTHY VEGETABLE FRIED RICE

**VEGETARIAN**
**30-MINUTE**
**BUDGET-SAVER**

**PREP** 5 minutes
**COOK** 10 minutes

**FOR THE SAUCE**

⅓ cup garlic vinegar

1½ tablespoons dark molasses

1 teaspoon onion powder

**FOR THE FRIED RICE**

1 teaspoon olive oil

2 whole eggs plus 4 egg whites, lightly beaten

1 cup frozen mixed vegetables

1 cup frozen edamame

2 cups cooked brown rice

*serves 4* **Even if you are actively managing a health condition, eating should be pleasurable, and there is no reason to feel deprived on the DASH eating plan. This recipe proves that you can enjoy your favorites like fried rice, which with some minor adjustments, will boost your nutrition intake and keep calories and sodium in check. Enjoy this lightened-up version of a popular takeout favorite.**

**TO MAKE THE SAUCE**

Prepare the sauce by combining the garlic vinegar, molasses, and onion powder in a glass jar. Shake well.

**TO MAKE THE FRIED RICE**

1. Heat oil in a large wok or skillet over medium-high heat. Add eggs and egg whites, let cook until the eggs set, for about 1 minute. Break up eggs with a spatula or spoon into small pieces. Add frozen mixed vegetables and frozen edamame. Cook for 4 minutes, stirring frequently.

2. Add the brown rice and sauce to the vegetable-and-egg mixture. Cook for 5 minutes or until heated through.

3. Serve immediately.

**INGREDIENT TIP** Edamame are easy to find and are located in the freezer section of the grocery store. High in complete high-quality plant-based protein and fiber, edamame are simply green soybeans. Choose the unshelled variety.

**Per Serving** Total Calories: 210; Total Fat: 6g; Saturated Fat: 1g; Cholesterol: 93mg; Sodium: 113mg; Potassium: 183mg; Total Carbohydrate: 28g; Fiber: 3g; Sugars: 6g; Protein: 13g

# PORTOBELLO-MUSHROOM CHEESEBURGERS

**VEGETARIAN**
**30-MINUTE**
**BUDGET-SAVER**

**PREP** 5 minutes
**COOK** 10 minutes

4 portobello mushrooms, caps removed and brushed clean

1 tablespoon olive oil

½ teaspoon freshly ground black pepper

1 tablespoon red wine vinegar

4 slices reduced-fat Swiss cheese, sliced thin

4 whole-wheat 100-calorie sandwich thins

½ avocado, sliced thin

*serves 4* An easy way to make your diet more nutrient dense is to serve up meatless meals once or twice a week. That's where these easy, and surprisingly meaty, Portobello cheeseburgers come in. Though very low in calories, a single cap of this mushroom has as much blood-pressure-regulating potassium as a banana, along with high amounts of filling fiber and B vitamins. Ready in just 10 minutes, top this meaty "burger" with your favorite fixings.

1. Heat a skillet or grill pan over medium-high heat. Clean the mushrooms and remove the stems. Brush each cap with olive oil and sprinkle with black pepper. Place in skillet cap-side up and cook for about 4 minutes. Flip and cook for another 4 minutes.

2. Sprinkle with the red wine vinegar and flip. Add the cheese and cook for 2 more minutes. For optimal melting, place a lid loosely over the pan.

3. Meanwhile, toast the sandwich thins. Create your burgers by topping each with sliced avocado.

4. Enjoy immediately.

**SUBSTITUTION TIP** You can find very thinly sliced whole-grain sandwich thins that would help you meet your whole-grain recommendations for the day. You could also opt to skip the buns and serve the burgers open-face style over a bed of fresh spinach.

**Per Serving** Total Calories: 245; Total Fat: 12g; Saturated Fat: 3g; Cholesterol: 15mg; Sodium: 266mg; Potassium: 507mg; Total Carbohydrate: 28g; Fiber: 8g; Sugars: 4g; Protein: 14g

# BAKED CHICKPEA-AND-ROSEMARY OMELET

**PREP** 10 minutes
**COOK** 15 minutes

½ tablespoon olive oil

4 eggs

¼ cup grated
Parmesan cheese

1 (15-ounce) can chickpeas,
drained and rinsed

2 cups packed baby spinach

1 cup button
mushrooms, chopped

2 sprigs rosemary, leaves
picked (or 2 teaspoons dried
rosemary)

Salt

Freshly ground black pepper

*serves 2* **Simple, satisfying, and quick to prepare, this recipe helps you meet your goals for protein, calcium, potassium, and magnesium.**

1. Preheat the oven to 400°F and place a baking tray on the middle shelf.

2. Line an 8-inch springform pan with baking paper and grease generously with olive oil. If you don't have a spring-form pan, grease an oven-safe skillet (or cast-iron skillet) with olive oil.

3. Lightly whisk together the eggs and Parmesan.

4. Place chickpeas in the prepared pan. Layer the spinach and mushrooms on top of the beans. Pour the egg mixture on top and scatter the rosemary. Season to taste with salt and pepper.

5. Place the pan on the preheated tray and bake until golden and puffy and the center feels firm and springy, about 15 minutes.

6. Remove from the oven, slice, and serve immediately.

**SUBSTITUTION TIP** You can vary the beans, vegetables, and cheese in this recipe and come up with your own favorite combinations. Try asparagus, goat cheese, and white beans for a delicious variation.

**Per Serving** Total Calories: 418; Total Fat: 19g; Saturated Fat: 6g; Cholesterol: 382mg; Sodium: 595mg; Potassium: 273mg; Total Carbohydrate: 33g; Fiber: 12g; Sugars: 2g; Protein: 30g

# CHILLED CUCUMBER-AND-AVOCADO SOUP WITH DILL

**VEGETARIAN**
**ONE POT**

**PREP** 5 minutes
**CHILL** 30 minutes

2 English cucumbers, peeled and diced, plus ¼ cup reserved for garnish

1 avocado, peeled, pitted, and diced, plus ¼ cup reserved for garnish

1½ cups nonfat or low-fat plain Greek yogurt

½ cup cold water

⅓ cup loosely packed dill, plus sprigs for garnish

1 tablespoon freshly squeezed lemon juice

¼ teaspoon freshly ground black pepper

¼ teaspoon salt

1 clove garlic

*serves 4* This refreshing chilled soup comes together in minutes without you ever having to turn on your cooktop. The smooth and creamy texture of avocado and Greek yogurt gives this soup a thick consistency without the heaviness of unhealthy sour cream. With high amounts of blood-pressure-lowering nutrients, including calcium and potassium, this soup is also rich in heart-healthy fats and filling fiber.

1. Purée ingredients in a blender until smooth. If you prefer a thinner soup, add more water until you reach the desired consistency.

2. Divide soup among 4 bowls. Cover with plastic wrap and refrigerate for 30 minutes.

3. Garnish with cucumber, avocado, and dill sprigs, if desired.

**BUDGET-SAVER TIP** English cucumbers are typically longer than regular cucumbers, contain fewer noticeable seeds, have a thinner skin, and have a milder flavor. However, they do cost more than garden cucumbers, but since this soup is puréed, the taste difference will be negligible. Simply adjust your seasonings.

**Per Serving** Total Calories: 142; Total Fat: 7g; Saturated Fat: 1g; Cholesterol: 4mg; Sodium: 193mg; Potassium: 421mg; Total Carbohydrate: 12g; Fiber: 4g; Sugars: 7g; Protein: 11g

# EASY CHICKPEA VEGGIE BURGERS

**VEGETARIAN**
**BUDGET-SAVER**

**PREP**: 10 minutes
**COOK**: 20 minutes

1 15-ounce can chickpeas, drained and rinsed

½ cup frozen spinach, thawed

⅓ cup rolled oats

1 teaspoon garlic powder

1 teaspoon onion powder

*serves 4* You don't have to be a vegetarian to enjoy veggie burgers! Homemade veggie burgers are easy to make and much more nutritious than the processed variety. Plus they make an economical meal and they freeze well, so you can have some on hand for later, too. This recipe uses chickpeas and spinach for a potassium- and fiber-rich burger, but your imagination is the only limit to the types of beans, seasonings, and veggies you can use.

1. Preheat oven to 400°F. Grease a cookie sheet or line one with parchment paper and set aside.

2. In a mixing bowl, add half of the beans and mash with a fork until mostly smooth. Set aside.

3. Add the remaining half of the beans, spinach, oats, and spices to a food processor or blender and blend until puréed. Add the mixture to the bowl of mashed beans and stir until well combined.

4. Divide mixture into 4 equal portions and shape into patties. Bake for 7 to 10 minutes, carefully flip over and bake for another 7 to 10 minutes, or until crusty on the outside.

5. Place on a whole grain bun with your favorite toppings.

**BUDGET-SAVER TIP** Use whatever vegetables you have on hand, which is a great way to utilize random veggie scraps instead of letting them go to waste. Mushrooms are excellent in veggie burgers, so are shredded carrots, shredded zucchini, and eggplant. Experiment until you get your favorite combination.

---

**Per Serving** Total Calories: 118; Total Fat: 1g; Saturated Fat: 0g; Cholesterol: 7mg; Sodium: 108mg; Potassium: 83mg; Total Carbohydrate: 21g; Fiber: 7g; Sugars: 0g; Protein: 7g

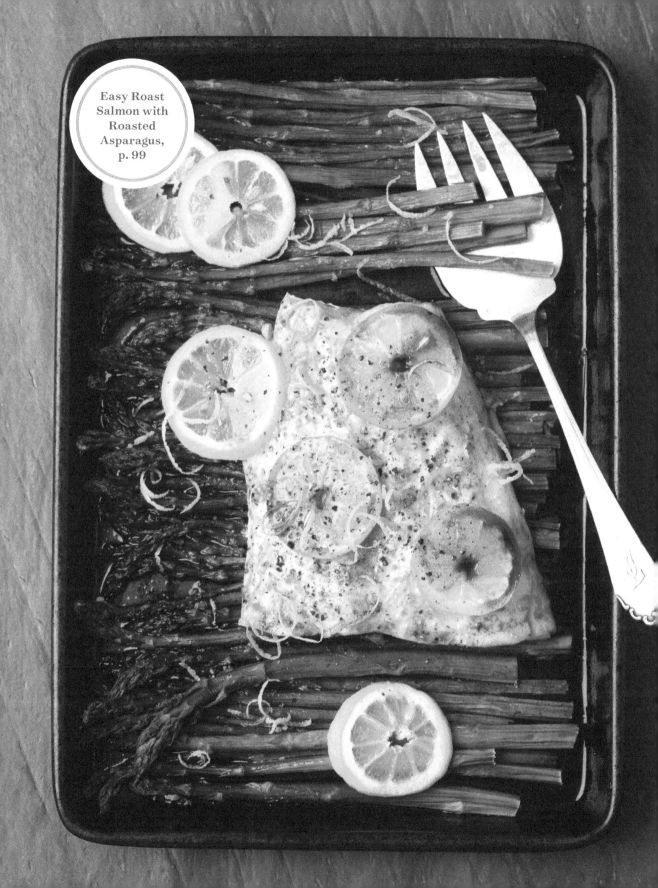

Easy Roast Salmon with Roasted Asparagus, p. 99

*seven*

# Poultry & Seafood Mains

Chicken and Broccoli Stir-Fry 92

Quick Chicken Fajitas 93

Honey-Mustard Chicken 94

Grilled Chicken, Avocado, and Apple Salad 95

Turkey Cutlets with Herbs 96

Balsamic-Roasted Chicken Breasts 97

Open-Faced Turkey Burger 98

Easy Roast Salmon with Roasted Asparagus 99

Shrimp Pasta Primavera 100

Cilantro-Lime Tilapia Tacos 101

Lemon-Parsley Baked Flounder and Brussels Sprouts 102

Pan-Seared Scallops 103

Baked Cod Packets with Broccoli and Squash 104

Garlic Salmon and Snap Peas in Foil 105

Salmon, Spinach, and Tomato Lasagna 106

Crispy Almond Chicken 107

# CHICKEN AND BROCCOLI STIR-FRY

**30-MINUTE**
**ONE POT**
**BUDGET-SAVER**

**PREP** 10 minutes
**COOK** 15 minutes

2 tablespoons sesame oil
(or olive oil), divided

2 boneless, skinless chicken
breasts, cubed

2 garlic cloves, minced

3 small carrots, thinly sliced

15 ounces frozen chopped
broccoli florets, thawed

8 ounces sliced water
chestnuts, drained and
thoroughly rinsed

3 tablespoons balsamic
vinegar, divided

2 teaspoons ground ginger

*serves 4* Stir-frying—cooking quickly over high heat—is a fast and fresh way to cook a simple dish of meat and vegetables. The shape of a wok, with its high sides, increases the amount of cooking surface you have—but if you don't own a wok you could also use a flat-bottom sauté pan. This quick and easy dish has all the flavor of your favorite takeout with far less sodium.

1. Heat ½ tablespoon of olive oil in a wok or large sauté pan over medium heat. Add the cubed chicken and cook until lightly browned and cooked through, about 5 to 7 minutes. Transfer chicken to a bowl, cover, and set aside.

2. Add 1½ tablespoons of olive oil to the pan, along with the garlic and carrots. Cook until the carrots begin to soften, about 3 to 4 minutes. Add the thawed broccoli florets and water chestnuts along with 1 tablespoon of balsamic vinegar and cook for 3 to 4 minutes.

3. Add the remaining balsamic vinegar and ground ginger. Add the cooked chicken back in and stir until well combined.

4. Serve over brown rice, if desired.

**INGREDIENT TIP** Even low-sodium soy sauce has about 500 milligrams of sodium in 1 tablespoon. Eliminate it from stir-fries and make up the flavor with vinegar and spices like ginger. Red wine vinegar goes well with beef, rice wine pairs well with vegetables, and balsamic nicely compliments chicken. Add some hot sauce, whose heat can mask the missing salty flavor.

**Per Serving** Total Calories: 189; Total Fat: 9g; Saturated Fat: 2g; Cholesterol: 33mg; Sodium: 68mg; Potassium: 228mg; Total Carbohydrate: 12g; Fiber: 3g; Sugars: 3g; Protein: 14g

# QUICK CHICKEN FAJITAS

30-MINUTE
ONE POT
BUDGET-SAVER

**PREP** 10 minutes
**COOK** 15 minutes

Cooking spray

4 cups frozen bell pepper strips

2 cups onion, sliced

1 pound boneless, skinless chicken breast, cut into thin slices

1 teaspoon ground cumin

1 teaspoon chili powder

2 (10-ounce) cans no-salt diced tomatoes and green chilies (Ro-Tel brand)

8 (6-inch) whole-wheat flour tortillas, warmed

*serves 4* **This simple and quick fajita recipe makes use of budget-conscious ingredients including frozen peppers and canned tomatoes— and both vegetables have high amounts of blood-pressure-lowering potassium. High in lean protein, this recipe makes a speedy weeknight meal.**

1. Spray a large skillet with cooking spray; heat over medium-high heat. Add the bell peppers and onions and cook for 7 minutes or until tender, stirring occasionally. Remove from skillet and set aside.

2. Add chicken to skillet. Sprinkle with cumin and chili powder. Cook for 4 minutes until no longer pink and an instant-read thermometer registers 165°F.

3. Return peppers and onions to skillet; add drained tomatoes and green chilies. Cook for 2 minutes more or until hot.

4. Divide mixture evenly between tortillas and serve immediately.

**INGREDIENT TIP** Available at most grocery stores, Ro-Tel sells canned no-salt-added diced tomatoes with green chilies. You could also use fresh tomatoes depending on cost and availability.

**Per Serving** Total Calories: 424; Total Fat: 8g; Saturated Fat: 2g; Cholesterol: 65mg; Sodium: 622mg; Potassium: 138mg; Total Carbohydrate: 51g; Fiber: 26g; Sugars: 5g; Protein: 33g

# HONEY-MUSTARD CHICKEN

**30-MINUTE**

**PREP** 5 minutes
**COOK** 15 minutes

¼ cup honey

¼ cup yellow mustard

¼ cup Dijon mustard

1 tablespoon olive oil

1 pound boneless, skinless chicken breasts

3 cups broccoli florets

½ teaspoon freshly ground black pepper

**BUDGET-SAVER TIP** Boneless, skinless chicken thighs also work well in this recipe, but you could also use bone-in, if you prefer. For the healthiest dish, always choose skinless chicken.

*serves 4* This super easy and quick recipe is loaded with flavor and delivers protein and vegetables in one skillet. The honey mustard coats the chicken and clings to the nooks and crannies of the broccoli, keeping it tender. Broccoli is a good source of magnesium and potassium and a very good source of filling dietary fiber. This dish is sure to hit the spot.

1. To a medium bowl, add the honey, yellow mustard, and Dijon mustard, whisk to combine, and taste to check for flavor balance, adding more honey and mustard if necessary. Set aside.

2. To a large skillet, add the oil and chicken and cook over medium-high heat for 3 to 5 minutes, then flip and cook for an additional 3 to 5 minutes. Cooking time will vary depending on the thickness of the chicken. Chicken should be almost cooked through.

3. Evenly drizzle the honey mustard over the chicken and flip each piece over a few times to ensure both sides are evenly coated.

4. Add the broccoli and stir to combine, making sure the broccoli gets coated with honey mustard. Cover and cook over medium-low heat, allowing the broccoli to steam for about 3 to 5 minutes or until broccoli is crisp tender and chicken is cooked through and an instant-read thermometer registers 165°F.

5. Serve immediately.

***

**Per Serving** Total Calories: 254; Total Fat: 8g; Saturated Fat: 2g; Cholesterol: 65mg; Sodium: 584mg; Potassium: 229mg; Total Carbohydrate: 21g; Fiber: 2g; Sugars: 17g; Protein: 27g

# GRILLED CHICKEN, AVOCADO, AND APPLE SALAD

**30-MINUTE**

**PREP** 15 minutes
**COOK** 8 minutes

Cooking spray

2 tablespoons olive oil

3 tablespoons balsamic vinegar

4 (4-ounce) skinless, boneless chicken-breast halves

8 cups mixed salad greens

1 cup diced peeled apple

¾ cup avocado, peeled and pitted

*Optional:* 2 tablespoons freshly squeezed lime juice

*serves 4* **This grilled-chicken salad is the perfect quick and easy dinner choice for a busy weeknight. Wonderfully refreshing and healthy, apples and avocado provide cholesterol-lowering fiber, while the greens add magnesium and calcium. Full of lean protein and flavor, this salad will satisfy your taste buds while giving you the nutrition you need.**

1. Prepare a grill for high heat. Apply cooking spray to the grill rack. If you don't have a grill, you can broil the chicken in an oven-safe skillet under the broiler element for 5 to 6 minutes.

2. Combine olive oil, balsamic vinegar, and lime juice (if using) in a small bowl. Place chicken on a large plate. Spoon 2 tablespoons of oil mixture over the chicken, reserving the rest for the salad dressing. Turn chicken to coat, and let stand for 5 minutes.

3. Place chicken on grill rack. Cook for 4 minutes on each side or until an instant-read thermometer registers 165°F. Remove to a plate and cut crosswise into strips.

4. Arrange greens, apple, and avocado on 4 serving plates. Arrange chicken over greens. Drizzle reserved dressing over salads.

> **BUDGET-SAVER TIP** If pre-washed baby salad greens are not in your budget, simply purchase a head or two of red- or green-leaf lettuce or bunches of fresh spinach. Be sure to wash and dry these before using. Avoid purchasing iceberg lettuce, as it is low in nutrients compared to other greens.

**Per Serving** Total Calories: 288; Total Fat: 16g; Saturated Fat: 3g; Cholesterol: 65mg; Sodium: 81mg; Potassium: 175mg; Total Carbohydrate: 8g; Fiber: 5g; Sugars: 4g; Protein: 27g

# TURKEY CUTLETS WITH HERBS

**30-MINUTE**
**ONE POT**
**BUDGET-SAVER**

**PREP** 5 minutes
**COOK** 8 minutes

2 tablespoons olive oil

2 lemons, sliced

1 package (approximately
1 pound) turkey-breast
cutlets (without antibiotics)

½ teaspoon garlic powder

Freshly ground black pepper

4 cups baby spinach

½ cup water

2 teaspoons dried thyme

*serves 4* This fast and flavorful recipe is great for a weeknight dinner. The entire dish cooks up in minutes using just one pan and a handful of ingredients. Turkey breast is an excellent lean protein and a good source of heart-healthy B vitamins and potassium. Not just for Thanksgiving, turkey-breast cutlets make a nutritious choice any time of year.

1. In a large skillet over medium-high heat, heat the oil.

2. Add about 6 lemon slices to the skillet.

3. Sprinkle the turkey-breast cutlets with garlic powder and black pepper. Place the turkey cutlets into the skillet and cook for about 3 minutes on each side until the turkey is no longer pink, and is slightly browned at the edges. Remove them from the heat and add them to 4 plates.

4. Add the spinach to the pan along with ½ cup of water and steam, stirring frequently for about 2 minutes. Remove the greens and lemons with tongs or a slotted spoon and divide between plates.

5. Serve topped with dried thyme.

**INGREDIENT TIP** Herbs and spices offer a number of health benefits as they are rich sources of vitamins and minerals. Thyme is a good source of the antioxidant vitamin C and disease-protective flavonoids. Dried herbs are more potent than fresh, so you need to use less—as a general rule, 1 teaspoon of dried herbs equals 1 tablespoon of fresh ones.

**Per Serving** Total Calories: 204; Total Fat: 8g; Saturated Fat: 1g; Cholesterol: 70mg; Sodium: 92mg; Potassium: 82mg; Total Carbohydrate: 8g; Fiber: 4g; Sugars: 1g; Protein: 30g

# BALSAMIC-ROASTED CHICKEN BREASTS

ONE POT

**PREP** 35 minutes
**COOK** 40 minutes

¼ cup balsamic vinegar

1 tablespoon olive oil

2 teaspoons dried oregano

2 garlic cloves, minced

⅛ teaspoon salt

½ teaspoon freshly ground black pepper

2 (4-ounce) boneless, skinless, chicken-breast halves

Cooking spray

*serves 2* **Baked balsamic chicken is wholesome, delicious, and very easy to make. Marinating the chicken breasts makes the meat extra tender and juicy. You can customize the recipe to use whatever herbs you have on hand. A good source of lean protein, chicken breast is very low in calories and is a good source of B vitamins, which are important for heart health.**

1. In a small bowl, add the vinegar, olive oil, oregano, garlic, salt, and pepper. Mix to combine.

2. Put the chicken in a resealable plastic bag. Pour the vinegar mixture in the bag with the chicken, seal the bag, and coat the chicken to marinate. Refrigerate for 30 minutes.

3. Preheat the oven to 400°F. Spray a small baking dish with cooking spray.

4. Put the chicken in prepared baking dish and pour the marinade over the chicken. Cover and bake for 35 to 40 minutes, or until an instant-read thermometer registers 165°F.

5. Let sit for 5 minutes, then serve with your favorite vegetables.

**BUDGET-SAVER TIP** Quick-cooking grain medleys are a healthy choice that make it easy and budget friendly to increase your consumption of whole grains. Several brands offer brown-rice and whole-grain medleys that can be prepared in just 10 minutes.

**Per Serving** Total Calories: 226; Total Fat: 11g; Saturated Fat: 3g; Cholesterol: 65mg; Sodium: 129mg; Potassium: 44mg; Total Carbohydrate: 6g; Fiber: 1g; Sugars: 0g; Protein: 25g

# OPEN-FACED TURKEY BURGER

**BUDGET-SAVER**

**PREP** 10 minutes
**COOK** 25 minutes

1 tablespoon olive oil

1 cup mushrooms, finely chopped

1 clove garlic, minced

1 pound lean ground white meat turkey

½ teaspoon freshly ground black pepper

⅛ teaspoon salt

Cooking spray

4 cups baby spinach

2 tomatoes, sliced

**INGREDIENT TIP** Shredded zucchini can be added to the skillet with the mushrooms and mixed in with the ground meat. Zucchini has a high water content so it can help the burgers stay moist and juicy. It will also boost the amount of fiber and servings of veggies in the meal.

*serves 4* **The DASH diet recommends you limit your consumption of red meats due to their high saturated-fat content. But that doesn't mean you need to give up burgers. Instead, this recipe replaces ground beef with leaner ground white turkey meat. Served over a bed of calcium-rich spinach and topped with potassium-rich tomatoes, this dish is filling and helps you meet your daily nutrient goals.**

1. Heat the olive oil in a skillet over medium-low heat. Add the mushrooms and cook until soft and browned, about 5 minutes. Add the garlic and cook for 1 additional minute. Turn off the heat and allow to cool slightly.

2. Add the turkey in a large bowl and add the mushroom-garlic mixture, pepper, and salt. Mix until well combined and form into 8 small patties.

3. Prepare a grill for medium-high heat. Apply cooking spray to the grill rack. Grill the burgers until cooked through, 6 to 8 minutes per side and until an instant-read thermometer registers 165°F. If you don't have a grill, you can broil the burgers in an oven-safe skillet under the broiler element for about 10 minutes per side, or until an instant-read thermometer registers 165°F.

4. Divide the spinach among 4 serving plates, top with 2 patties per plate. Add tomato slices and serve immediately.

**Per Serving** Total Calories: 179; Total Fat: 5g; Saturated Fat: 1g; Cholesterol: 55mg; Sodium: 135mg; Potassium: 198mg; Total Carbohydrate: 6g; Fiber: 2g; Sugars: 1g; Protein: 28g

# EASY ROAST SALMON WITH ROASTED ASPARAGUS

**30-MINUTE**
**ONE POT**

**PREP** 5 minutes
**COOK** 15 minutes

2 (5-ounce) salmon fillets with skin

2 teaspoons olive oil, plus extra for drizzling

Salt

Freshly ground black pepper

1 bunch asparagus, trimmed

1 teaspoon dried chives

1 teaspoon dried tarragon

Fresh lemon wedges for serving

*serves 2* **Salmon is an excellent source of heart-healthy omega-3 fatty acids—for optimum health, recommendations are to include at least 2 servings of salmon or another fatty fish each week. This recipe is easy and fancy—a perfect dish for any night of the week.**

1. Preheat the oven to 425°F.

2. Rub salmon all over with 1 teaspoon of olive oil per fillet. Season with salt and pepper.

3. Place asparagus spears on a foil lined baking sheet and lay the salmon fillets skin-side down on top. Put pan in upper-third of oven and roast until fish is just cooked through, about 12 minutes. Roasting time will vary depending on the thickness of your salmon. Salmon should flake easily with a fork when it's ready and an instant-read thermometer should register 145°F.

4. When cooked, remove from the oven, cut fillets in half crosswise, then lift flesh from skin with a metal spatula and transfer to a plate. Discard the skin, then drizzle salmon with oil, sprinkle with herbs, and serve with lemon wedges and roasted asparagus spears.

**BUDGET-SAVER TIP** There is a wide range of price, color, and taste among the six species of salmon we commonly eat, so as with any fish, buy the best salmon you can find and afford. Pink and chum are smaller fish and are good budget choices.

**Per Serving** Total Calories: 353; Total Fat: 22g; Saturated Fat: 4g; Cholesterol: 88mg; Sodium: 90mg; Potassium: 304mg; Total Carbohydrate: 5g; Fiber: 2g; Sugars: 0g; Protein: 34g

# SHRIMP PASTA PRIMAVERA

30-MINUTE
ONE POT

PREP 5 minutes
COOK 15 minutes

2 tablespoons olive oil

1 tablespoon garlic, minced

2 cups assorted fresh vegetables, chopped coarsely (zucchini, broccoli, asparagus, whatever you prefer)

4 ounces frozen shrimp, cooked, peeled, and deveined

Salt

Freshly ground black pepper

Juice of ½ lemon

4 ounces whole-wheat angel-hair pasta, cooked per package instructions

2 tablespoons grated Parmesan cheese

*serves 2* **This low-calorie, well-seasoned, flavorful pasta dish comes together in just minutes and is easy on the budget. Shrimp are low in calories and are protein-rich—and while they do contain cholesterol, dietary cholesterol has a minimal impact on blood cholesterol.** *Primavera* **in Italian means "spring," as in a "mixture of fresh spring vegetables," so feel free to use your favorites to customize this recipe.**

1. Heat the oil in a large nonstick skillet over medium heat. Add the garlic and sauté for 1 minute.

2. Add vegetables and sauté until crisp tender, 3 to 4 minutes.

3. Add the shrimp and sauté until just heated through. Season lightly with salt and pepper and squeeze lemon juice over the shrimp and vegetables. Continue to cook for about 2 minutes until the juices have been reduced by about half. Remove from heat.

4. Toss shrimp and vegetables with pasta. Serve topped with Parmesan cheese.

**BUDGET-SAVER TIP** You can cut down on cost by replacing the fresh vegetables with a 16-ounce bag of frozen mixed vegetables. Read the ingredients list and make sure that there is no added salt or seasonings.

**Per Serving** Total Calories: 439; Total Fat: 17g; Saturated Fat: 3g; Cholesterol: 105mg; Sodium: 286mg; Potassium: 481mg; Total Carbohydrate: 50g; Fiber: 8g; Sugars: 5g; Protein: 23g

# CILANTRO-LIME TILAPIA TACOS

**30-MINUTE**

**PREP** 10 minutes
**COOK** 10 minutes

1 teaspoon olive oil

1 pound tilapia fillets, rinsed and dried

3 cups diced tomatoes

½ cup fresh cilantro, chopped, plus additional for serving

3 tablespoons freshly squeezed lime juice

Salt

Freshly ground black pepper

8 (5-inch) white-corn tortillas

1 avocado sliced into 8 wedges

*Optional:* lime wedges and fat-free sour cream for serving

*serves 4* These fish tacos are a refreshing, light meal—offering a good source of lean, high-quality protein. High in potassium from the vegetable mix and low in sodium, simply add a glass of low-fat milk and fruit for dessert for a complete meal rich in blood-pressure-lowering nutrients.

1. Heat the oil in a large skillet, add the tilapia and cook until the flesh starts to flake, about 5 minutes per side.

2. Add the tomatoes, cilantro, and lime juice. Sauté over medium-high heat for about 5 minutes, breaking up the fish to get everything mixed well. Season to taste with salt and pepper.

3. Meanwhile heat tortillas on a skillet for a few minutes on each side to warm.

4. Serve ¼ cup of fish mixture on each warmed tortilla with two slices of avocado.

5. Serve immediately with optional toppings, if using.

**INGREDIENT TIP** If you like your tacos spicy, add 1 to 2 seeded and chopped jalapeños when you add the tomatoes, cilantro, and lime juice. You could also add a few splashes of your favorite hot sauce instead.

**Per Serving** Total Calories: 286; Total Fat: 12g; Saturated Fat: 2g; Cholesterol: 55mg; Sodium: 117mg; Potassium: 860mg; Total Carbohydrate: 22g; Fiber: 4g; Sugars: 0g; Protein: 28g

# LEMON-PARSLEY BAKED FLOUNDER AND BRUSSELS SPROUTS

**30-MINUTE**

**PREP** 10 minutes
**COOK** 15 minutes

14 Brussels sprouts

2 tablespoons olive oil, divided

3 tablespoons freshly squeezed lemon juice

1 tablespoon minced fresh garlic

¼ teaspoon dried dill

2 (6-ounce) flounder fillets

Salt

Freshly ground black pepper

*serves 2* **Flounder and other white fish are very low in calories and fat and provide an excellent source of filling protein. And since DASH recommends increasing your intake of vegetables, this recipe makes use of oven time to roast a tray of potassium-rich Brussels sprouts.**

1. Preheat the oven to 400°F. Rinse the Brussels sprouts and pat them dry. Cut their stem ends off, then cut sprouts in half and place them on a foil-lined baking pan. Drizzle with 1 tablespoon olive oil and toss to coat.

2. Meanwhile in a small bowl, stir together 1 tablespoon olive oil, lemon juice, garlic, and dill.

3. Rinse flounder fillets and pat dry, season lightly with salt and pepper. Place in baking dish and evenly drizzle oil-and-herb mixture over flounder fillets.

4. Bake for 10 to 11 minutes, or until the fish flakes easily when tested with a fork. The Brussels sprouts should be lightly browned and also pierce easily with a fork.

5. Divide the flounder and Brussels sprouts between serving plates.

**INGREDIENT TIP** Roasting vegetables is easy to do and intensifies flavors. For best results, use a shallow pan and don't overcrowd it. Season them with olive oil and your favorite herbs.

**Per Serving** Total Calories: 319; Total Fat: 17g; Saturated Fat: 2g; Cholesterol: 98mg; Sodium: 529mg; Potassium: 538mg; Total Carbohydrate: 13g; Fiber: 5g; Sugars: 3g; Protein: 33g

# PAN-SEARED SCALLOPS

**30-MINUTE**
**ONE POT**

**PREP** 5 minutes
**COOK** 6 minutes

2 cups chopped tomato

½ cup chopped fresh basil

¼ teaspoon freshly ground black pepper, divided

2 tablespoons olive oil, divided

1½ pounds sea scallops

⅛ teaspoon salt

1 cup fresh corn kernels

1 cup zucchini, diced

*serves 4* **Scallops contain a variety of heart-health-promoting nutrients, including B vitamins, omega-3 fats, and the minerals magnesium and potassium. With a delicate, mild flavor, scallops are quick to prepare, low in calories, and rich in high-quality protein. This recipe comes together in minutes and makes use of fresh summer vegetables that pair nicely with the scallops.**

1. In a medium bowl, combine tomato, basil, and ⅛ teaspoon black pepper. Toss gently.

2. Heat a large skillet over high heat. Add 1 tablespoon of olive oil to the pan, swirling to coat. Pat scallops dry with paper towels. Sprinkle with salt and remaining black pepper. Add scallops to the pan, cook for 2 minutes or until browned. Turn scallops and cook for 2 minutes more or until browned. Remove scallops from the pan and keep warm.

3. Heat the remaining olive oil in the pan. Add corn and zucchini to the pan. Sauté for 2 minutes or until lightly browned. Add to tomato mixture and toss gently.

4. Serve scallops with a spinach salad, if desired.

**BUDGET-SAVER TIP** You can use frozen corn in place of fresh corn if it is not in season. You can also replace the fresh basil with 1 tablespoon of dried. Add 1 to 2 cups of fresh spinach to the salad in its place.

**Per Serving** Total Calories: 221; Total Fat: 9g; Saturated Fat: 1g; Cholesterol: 35mg; Sodium: 214mg; Potassium: 444mg; Total Carbohydrate: 17g; Fiber: 3g; Sugars: 5g; Protein: 20g

# BAKED COD PACKETS WITH BROCCOLI AND SQUASH

**30-MINUTE**
**SHEET PAN**

**PREP** 10 minutes
**COOK** 20 minutes

2 cups summer squash, sliced

2 cups small broccoli florets

4 garlic cloves, minced

2 tablespoons olive oil

Salt

Freshly ground black pepper

4 (4-ounce) cod fillets

4 teaspoons dried thyme

Juice of 1 lemon

**INGREDIENT TIP** While you can use any type of fresh or dried herb you like, some good choices for white fish include: parsley, cumin, oregano, basil, paprika, lemon zest, ginger, cayenne, garlic, onion, and coriander.

*serves 4* Wrapping fish and vegetables in a foil packet for baking is a very fast way to prepare a complete, nutrient-dense meal with no fuss and no cookware to wash. Sealing the fish and vegetables in foil steams the contents to enhance the flavors— a foolproof way to get moist and tender results. You can adapt this recipe according to which vegetables are in season and to whichever fish fits your budget.

1. Preheat the oven to 400°F. Cut aluminum foil into 4, 12-inch squares and arrange them on a work surface. Fold each piece in half to form a crease down the middle. Spray the foil with cooking spray.

2. Divide squash between the squares, arranging it just to the right of each crease. Top squash with broccoli and garlic, then drizzle with olive oil and sprinkle with salt and pepper.

3. Arrange 1 fillet on top of each pile of vegetables, then season fillets with salt and pepper. Top each fillet with 1 teaspoon of dried thyme.

4. Drizzle lemon juice over the fillets, then wrap each square of foil to form a sealed pouch. Transfer pouches to a baking sheet and bake until the fish is cooked through, about 20 minutes.

5. Set aside to rest for 3 to 4 minutes. Then cut pouches open, being careful of the steam, and serve immediately.

---

**Per Serving** Total Calories: 184; Total Fat: 8g; Saturated Fat: 1g; Cholesterol: 40mg; Sodium: 95mg; Potassium: 397mg; Total Carbohydrate: 8g; Fiber: 3g; Sugars: 2g; Protein: 22g

# GARLIC SALMON AND SNAP PEAS IN FOIL

**30-MINUTE**
**SHEET PAN**

**PREP** 5 minutes
**COOK** 15 minutes

Cooking spray

2 (4-ounce) skinless salmon fillets

2 cups sugar snap peas, divided

2 garlic cloves, minced and divided

Juice of 1 lemon, divided

Salt

Freshly ground black pepper

*serves 2* **If you are actively managing your weight, meals that provide ample amounts of protein and fiber are your best bet for keeping you feeling full and satisfied. In this simple and quick foil-packet recipe, omega-3-rich salmon provides high-quality protein with a dose of healthy fats, while sugar snap peas add fiber, the antioxidant vitamin C, and the DASH-recommended minerals potassium and magnesium. Ready in under 30 minutes, serve with a green salad and brown rice.**

1. Preheat the oven to 450°F.

2. Cut 2 large squares of aluminum foil, each about 12-by-18 inches. Spray the center of each foil sheet with cooking spray.

3. Place 1 salmon fillet in the center of each sheet, top with 1 cup of sugar snap peas, 1 clove minced garlic, and drizzle with lemon juice. Sprinkle with salt and pepper if desired.

4. Bring up the sides of the foil and fold top over twice.

5. Seal ends, leaving room for air to circulate inside the packet.

6. Place packets on a baking sheet and cook in oven for 15 to 18 minutes, or until salmon is opaque.

7. Use caution when opening the packets as the steam is very hot. Serve with lemon wedges on the side, if desired.

**INGREDIENT TIP** You can use your favorite vegetables in this recipe. Try it with the following when they are in season: asparagus, red bell peppers, mushrooms, summer squash, or even slices of eggplant.

**Per Serving** Total Calories: 211; Total Fat: 5g; Saturated Fat: 1g; Cholesterol: 50mg; Sodium: 86mg; Potassium: 41mg; Total Carbohydrate: 14g; Fiber: 3g; Sugars: 5g; Protein: 26g

# SALMON, SPINACH, AND TOMATO LASAGNA

**PREP** 30 minutes
**COOK** 1 hour

1½ cups white wine

2 garlic cloves,
slightly crushed

4 tablespoons fresh dill

¼ teaspoon salt

1 teaspoon freshly ground
black pepper

1 pound salmon fillet

16 ounces whole-wheat
lasagna noodles, cooked
al dente

1 cup baby spinach, divided

1 cup nonfat or low-fat plain
Greek yogurt, divided

2 cups partly skim mozzarella
cheese, shredded and divided

*serves 8–10* **This spin on traditional lasagna uses heart-healthy, omega-3 fatty acid–rich salmon and, for an additional nutrition boost, whole-wheat noodles. This beautiful dish is perfect for a family gathering or a special occasion. By cooking this impressive lasagna, you can wow your guests while staying true to your DASH diet. High in calcium, magnesium, and protein, this filling dish makes plenty of leftovers for freezing. Serve with a fresh green salad.**

1. Preheat the oven to 350°F. In a shallow saucepan, add wine, garlic, dill, and salt and pepper. Bring to a low simmer. Add salmon and poach until cooked, turning once. Allow to cool and set aside. Flake salmon into bite-size pieces. Refrigerate for 15 minutes.

2. Oil a 9-by-13-inch baking dish. Layer ⅓ pasta, spinach, salmon, Greek yogurt, and mozzarella cheese. Repeat layers 3 times, and make sure cheese is on top. Bake for 30 to 35 minutes until cheese is melted and golden brown.

3. Allow to cool for 5 to 10 minutes. Serve.

**SUBSTITUTION TIP** Regular Greek yogurt is used in place of crème fraîche in this recipe in order to reduce the amount of saturated fat. However, feel free to purchase crème fraîche and make the ingredient substitution.

**Per Serving** Total Calories: 385; Total Fat: 9g; Saturated Fat: 4g; Cholesterol: 44mg; Sodium: 310mg; Potassium: 10mg; Total Carbohydrate: 46g; Fiber: 6g; Sugars: 2g; Protein: 29g

# CRISPY ALMOND CHICKEN

**BUDGET SAVER**

**PREP** 10 minutes
**COOK** 25 minutes

½ cup almond meal

1 teaspoon ground paprika

½ teaspoon black pepper

⅛ teaspoon salt

4 4-ounce boneless, skinless chicken breasts

*serves 4* **This quick and easy recipe is a healthy version of "shake and bake" chicken. Heart healthy almond meal is used in this recipe, making it a perfect dish for everyone—including those following a gluten-free diet. A great go-to recipe when you are in a hurry, the coating ensures the chicken is always extra juicy.**

1. Preheat oven to 350°F.

2. Combine almond meal, paprika, salt, and pepper in a resealable bag. Put each chicken breast in the bag one at a time; close bag and shake until evenly coated. Place chicken in glass baking dish.

3. Bake in the preheated oven until no longer pink in the middle and juices run clear, 25 to 30 minutes. An instant-read thermometer inserted into the center should read 165°F.

4. Serve with a fresh green salad and your favorite sides.

BUDGET SAVER TIP You can also make this with recipe with boneless, skinless chicken thighs.

**Per Serving** Total Calories: 222; Total Fat: 11g; Saturated Fat: 2g; Cholesterol: 65mg; Sodium: 79mg; Potassium: 16mg; Total Carbohydrate: 3g; Fiber: 2g; Sugars: 1g; Protein: 28g

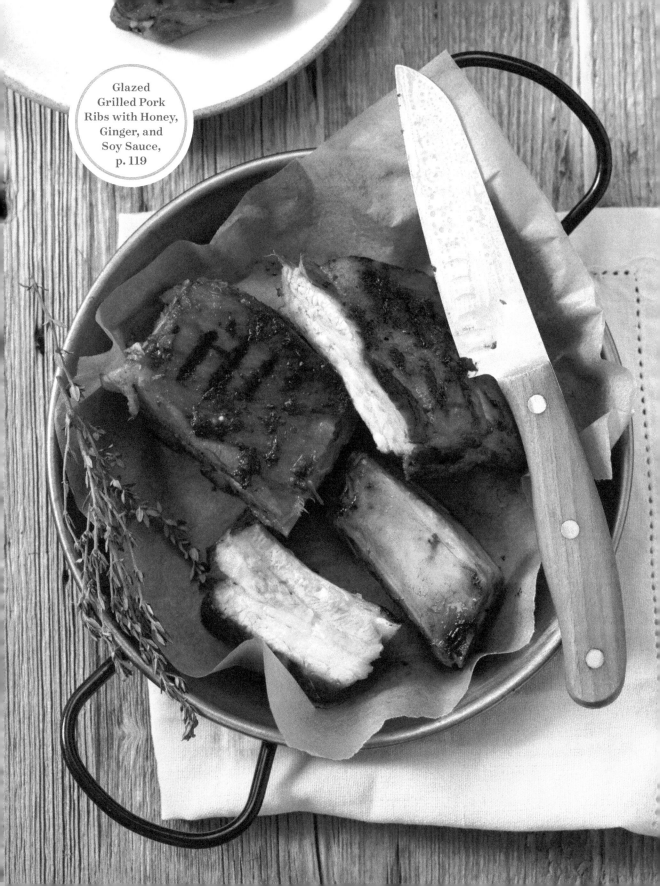

Glazed Grilled Pork Ribs with Honey, Ginger, and Soy Sauce, p. 119

# *eight*
# Beef & Pork Mains

Mustard-Crusted Pork
Tenderloin **110**

Apple-Cinnamon Baked
Pork Chops **111**

Pork Medallions with
Spring Succotash **112**

Pork Salad with Walnuts
and Peaches **113**

Pork, White Bean,
and Spinach Soup **114**

Orange-Beef Stir-Fry **115**

Steak Tacos **116**

Grilled Steak, Onions,
and Mushrooms **117**

Beef-and-Bean Chili **118**

Glazed Grilled Pork
Ribs with Honey, Ginger,
and Soy Sauce **119**

# MUSTARD-CRUSTED PORK TENDERLOIN

30-MINUTE
ONE POT

**PREP** 15 minutes
**COOK** 15 minutes

3 tablespoons Dijon mustard

3 tablespoons honey

1 teaspoon dried rosemary

1 tablespoon olive oil

1 pound pork tenderloin

Salt

Freshly ground black pepper

*serves 4* **Technically a type of red meat, certain cuts of pork are very lean and low in fat. Pork tenderloin is one of the most tender cuts of pork, and it is easy to cook. This recipe uses a mustard coating for a juicy result. Serve this dish with a side of steamed vegetables and fresh green salad.**

1. Preheat the oven to 425°F with the rack set in the middle. In a small bowl, combine the Dijon mustard, honey, and rosemary. Stir to combine, set aside.

2. Preheat an oven-safe skillet over high heat and add the olive oil. While it is heating up, pat pork loin dry with a paper towel and season lightly with salt and pepper on all sides. When the skillet is hot, sear the pork loin on all sides until golden brown, about 3 minutes per side. Remove from the heat and spread honey-mustard mixture evenly to coat the pork loin.

3. Place the skillet in the oven and cook the pork loin for 15 minutes, or until an instant-read thermometer registers 145°F.

4. Remove from the oven and allow to rest for 3 minutes. Slice the pork into ½-inch slices and serve.

**INGREDIENT TIP** Pork cooking-temperature guidelines have been revised in recent years because today's pork is more lean and safe. For best results, target an internal pork cooking temperature between 145°F and 160°F. Measure the temperature at the thickest part of the cut. Remember to allow the pork to rest for 3 minutes before serving.

**Per Serving** Total Calories: 220; Total Fat: 9g; Saturated Fat: 3g; Cholesterol: 45mg; Sodium: 307mg; Potassium: 11mg; Total Carbohydrate: 14g; Fiber: 0g; Sugars: 13g; Protein: 19g

# APPLE-CINNAMON BAKED PORK CHOPS

**ONE POT**

**PREP** 10 minutes
**COOK** 40 minutes

2 apples, peeled, cored, and sliced

1 teaspoon ground cinnamon, divided

4 boneless pork chops (½-inch thick)

Salt

Freshly ground black pepper

¾ cup water

3 tablespoons brown sugar

1 tablespoon olive oil

*serves 4* **This satisfying sweet and savory dish pairs simple ingredients and pantry staples to create a delicious flavor combination. Pork chops are a budget-friendly protein and apples are available year round, making this an inexpensive yet healthy dinner that can help you meet your fruit and protein servings for the day. Serve this dish with a side of steamed green beans.**

1. Preheat the oven to 375°F. Layer apples in bottom of casserole dish. Sprinkle with ½ teaspoon of cinnamon.

2. Trim fat from the pork chops. Lay chops on top of the apple slices. Sprinkle with a dash of salt and pepper.

3. In a small bowl, combine ¾ cup of water, brown sugar, and remaining cinnamon. Pour the mixture over the chops. Drizzle the chops with 1 tablespoon of olive oil.

4. Bake uncovered in preheated oven for 30 to 45 minutes or until an instant-read thermometer registers between 145°F and 160°F. Allow to rest for 3 minutes before serving.

**INGREDIENT TIP** To enhance the taste of this dish, substitute 100 percent apple juice or apple cider in place of the water. Be certain to read the ingredients list and choose a variety without added sugar.

**Per Serving** Total Calories: 244; Total Fat: 10g; Saturated Fat: 3g; Cholesterol: 45mg; Sodium: 254mg; Potassium: 124mg; Total Carbohydrate: 22g; Fiber: 4g; Sugars: 19g; Protein: 21g

# PORK MEDALLIONS WITH SPRING SUCCOTASH

30-MINUTE

**PREP** 10 minutes
**COOK** 20 minutes

1 pound pork tenderloin, trimmed and cut into 1-inch-thick slices

2 teaspoons minced garlic

1 teaspoon dried rosemary

1½ tablespoons olive oil, divided

1 cup low-sodium chicken stock

1 cup carrots, halved and thinly sliced

3 tablespoons water

½ teaspoon freshly ground black pepper

2 cups frozen lima beans, thawed

1 cup frozen spinach, thawed

**INGREDIENT TIP** For a higher-protein succotash variation, replace the lima beans with frozen shelled edamame. You might also double the succotash recipe and serve leftovers as a light lunch salad.

*serves 4* **A traditional Southern side dish, succotash is packed with lots of healthy vegetables that typically include corn, lima beans, and onions. In this version, starchy corn is replaced with lower-calorie, potassium- and magnesium-rich spinach, making for a delicious and filling heart-healthy meal.**

1. Gently pound pork slices to ½-inch-thick medallions with a meat mallet or the heel of your hand.

2. Combine garlic and rosemary in a small bowl.

3. Heat a large skillet over medium heat. Add 1 tablespoon of olive oil and swirl to coat. Add the pork to the pan and cook for 4 minutes without turning. Turn and cook for 3 minutes or until desired degree of doneness. Remove pork from pan and keep warm.

4. Add garlic mixture; sauté for 1 minute or until fragrant. Add chicken stock and cook for 30 seconds or until reduced to ½ cup. Remove pan from heat.

5. Heat a second large nonstick skillet over medium heat. Add remaining olive oil and swirl to coat. Add carrots and cook for 2 minutes. Stir in water and black pepper. Cover and cook for 2 minutes until carrots are crisp tender. Stir in lima beans and spinach, cook for 3 minutes or until thoroughly heated.

6. Divide vegetable mixture among 4 plates. Top each serving with pork and sauce.

**Per Serving** Total Calories: 317; Total Fat: 11g; Saturated Fat: 3g; Cholesterol: 45mg; Sodium: 150mg; Potassium: 626mg; Total Carbohydrate: 28g; Fiber: 8g; Sugars: 2g; Protein: 28g

# PORK SALAD WITH WALNUTS AND PEACHES

**30-MINUTE**
**ONE POT**

**PREP** 15 minutes
**COOK** 10 minutes

1 tablespoon olive oil

1 pound pork tenderloin, cut into 1-inch cubes

1 (10-ounce) bag fresh spinach leaves

1 peach, pitted and sliced

¼ cup walnuts

Balsamic vinegar

*serves 4* **Enjoying more salads is a great way to increase your intake of the minerals potassium and magnesium. Leafy greens are one of the top sources of these important blood-pressure-lowering minerals, especially dark leafy greens like spinach. With a healthy dose of lean, high-quality protein from pork, healthy fats from walnuts, and a fruit serving, too, this nutrient-dense salad is an excellent choice when watching your weight.**

1. Heat the olive oil in a large nonstick skillet over medium-high heat. Add the pork and cook until it is browned on the outside and cooked through, 3 to 4 minutes per side. Remove from heat and set aside.

2. Make a bed of spinach on each individual serving plate. Arrange peach slices over the spinach. Top with the cooked pork and sprinkle with walnuts. Drizzle balsamic vinegar over the salad.

3. Enjoy immediately.

**BUDGET-SAVER TIP** Here are three ways to further lower the cost of this recipe: (1) buy a bunch of spinach instead of a bag of pre-washed spinach, (2) use whatever fruit is in season in place of the peach (try a pear, apple, or citrus fruit for a tangy flavor variation), and (3) use boneless pork chops cut into bite-size pieces in place of pork tenderloin.

**Per Serving** Total Calories: 230; Total Fat: 14g; Saturated Fat: 3g; Cholesterol: 45mg; Sodium: 69mg; Potassium: 81mg; Total Carbohydrate: 6g; Fiber: 2g; Sugars: 2g; Protein: 21g

# PORK, WHITE BEAN, AND SPINACH SOUP

**30-MINUTE**
**ONE POT**

**PREP** 10 minutes
**COOK** 15 minutes

1 tablespoon olive oil

8 ounces pork tenderloin or boneless pork chops, cut into 1-inch cubes

Salt

4 garlic cloves, minced

2 teaspoons paprika

1 (14.5-ounce) can diced no-salt tomatoes

4 cups low-sodium chicken broth

1 bunch spinach, ribs removed and chopped, about 8 cups, lightly packed

2 (15-ounce) cans white beans, drained and rinsed

**BUDGET-SAVER TIP** If fresh spinach isn't in your budget, here is a rule of thumb you can use: 8 cups of lightly packed fresh spinach cooks down to about 1 cup. One 10-ounce package of frozen spinach yields about 1½ cups after cooking, which would make a perfect substitution in this recipe with the bonus of even more healthy minerals.

*serves 4* Having a few quick and easy soup recipes in your repertoire can help you stay on track with the DASH eating plan and can help you be successful at managing your weight. Soups don't have to be fancy, and depending on your preferences, you can add more or different types of vegetables. This satisfying recipe is full of filling protein, fiber-rich beans, and magnesium- and potassium-rich vegetables. Serve it with a glass of low-fat milk for a complete DASH meal.

1. Heat the oil in a Dutch oven or heavy-bottom pot over medium-high heat. Season pork with a pinch of salt. When the pan is hot, add pork and cook, stirring occasionally, for about 2 minutes, long enough to encourage a good sear and brown sides. Transfer to a plate.

2. In the same pot, add the garlic and paprika. Cook, stirring often, until fragrant, about 30 seconds. Add tomatoes and increase heat to high and stir to scrape down any browned bits. Add broth and bring to a boil.

3. Add spinach until it just wilts, about 2 to 3 minutes. Reduce heat to maintain a simmer, stir in the beans, reserved pork, and any accumulated juices; simmer until the beans and pork are heated through, about 2 minutes.

4. Serve immediately.

**Per Serving** Total Calories: 327; Total Fat: 8g; Saturated Fat: 2g; Cholesterol: 22mg; Sodium: 389mg; Potassium: 511mg; Total Carbohydrate: 41g; Fiber: 15g; Sugars: 5g; Protein: 26g

# ORANGE-BEEF STIR-FRY

**PREP** 10 minutes
**COOK** 10 minutes

1 tablespoon cornstarch

¼ cup cold water

¼ cup orange juice

1 tablespoon reduced-sodium soy sauce

½ pound boneless beef sirloin steak, cut into thin strips

2 teaspoons olive oil, divided

3 cups frozen stir-fry vegetable blend

1 garlic clove, minced

*serves 2* **This orange-beef stir-fry may just become one of your favorite go-to recipes when you need to put a healthy dinner on the table fast. Full of flavor and color, this 2-serving recipe will satisfy that craving for takeout in a healthy, DASH-friendly way. This dish is high in lean protein and vitamin- and mineral-rich vegetables, with a kick of spice from the red pepper flakes.**

1. In a small bowl, combine the cornstarch, cold water, orange juice, and soy sauce until smooth. Set aside.

2. In a large skillet or wok, stir-fry beef in 1 teaspoon of olive oil for 3 to 4 minutes or until no longer pink. Remove with a slotted spoon and keep warm.

3. Stir-fry the vegetable blend and garlic in the remaining oil for 3 minutes. Stir cornstarch mixture and add to the pan. Bring to a boil; cook and stir for 2 minutes or until thickened. Add the beef and heat through.

**BUDGET-SAVER TIP** Buy the amount of beef your budget allows. You can reduce the beef by half and add in 1 cup of frozen protein-rich edamame. This would also help you practice taking the focus off meat and making the meal more plant-based.

**Per Serving** Total Calories: 268; Total Fat: 10g; Saturated Fat: 3g; Cholesterol: 65mg; Sodium: 376mg; Potassium: 65mg; Total Carbohydrate: 8g; Fiber: 3g; Sugars: 8g; Protein: 26g

# STEAK TACOS

30-MINUTE
ONE POT

**PREP** 15 minutes
**COOK** 13 minutes

1 pound beef flank (or round) steak

1 teaspoon chili powder

1 teaspoon olive oil

1 green bell pepper, cored and coarsely chopped

1 red onion, coarsely chopped

8 (6-inch) corn tortillas, warm

2 tablespoons freshly squeezed lime juice

*Optional for serving:*
1 avocado, sliced, and coarsely chopped cilantro

*serves 4* These tasty tacos come together in minutes—featuring seasoned beef with a generous amount of vitamin-, mineral-, and fiber-rich sautéed vegetables (which are also low in calories). With an additional serving of fruit and heart-healthy fats from creamy avocado, steak lovers are in for a treat with this speedy recipe.

1. Rub the steak with chili powder (and salt and pepper, if desired).

2. Heat olive oil in a large skillet over medium-high heat.

3. Add steak and cook for 6 to 8 minutes on each side or until it reaches your desired degree of doneness. Remove from heat.

4. Place steak on a plate and cover with aluminum foil. Let rest for 5 minutes.

5. Add the bell pepper and onion to skillet. Cook on medium heat, stirring frequently, for 3 to 5 minutes or until onion is translucent. Remove from heat.

6. Cut steak against the grain into thin slices.

7. Top tortillas evenly with beef, onion mixture, and lime juice. Garnish with avocado and cilantro, if using.

8. Serve immediately.

**INGREDIENT TIP** Corn tortillas are very low in calories and are a surprisingly good source of the blood-pressure-lowering minerals calcium and potassium. If you are trying to lose weight, tortillas make a good bread replacement due to their lower calorie content.

**Per Serving** Total Calories: 358; Total Fat: 12g; Saturated Fat: 4g; Cholesterol: 40mg; Sodium: 139mg; Potassium: 503mg; Total Carbohydrate: 34g; Fiber: 2g; Sugars: 0g; Protein: 28g

# GRILLED STEAK, ONIONS, AND MUSHROOMS

**PREP** 5 minutes
**COOK** 25 minutes

1 tablespoon olive oil, plus enough for grill rack

2 (4-ounce) filet steaks (1½-inches thick)

Salt

Freshly ground black pepper

2 cups sliced mushrooms

1 cup sliced red onion

*serves 2* **This protein-packed dish is low in sodium and fat. It includes 3 servings of vegetables in each portion. Aim to limit your consumption of red meat to an occasional treat—and when you do choose red meat, fill half of your plate with vegetables, which is easy to do with this recipe.**

1. Prepare a grill for high heat. Apply olive oil to the grill rack.

2. Sprinkle steaks lightly with salt and pepper.

3. Place steaks on grill with direct high heat and sear for 1 to 2 minutes per side. Reduce heat to medium and cook for 18 to 23 minutes or until done according to your preference, turning once during cooking. Transfer steaks to a plate and cover with foil; let rest for 5 minutes before serving.

4. In a medium sauté pan, heat the oil over medium-high heat on the grill. Add mushrooms and onions and sauté for 5 to 6 minutes until tender.

5. Serve the steak with the mushrooms and onions and a fresh green salad.

**INGREDIENT TIP** You can also "grill" indoors by heating olive oil in a medium skillet over high heat, adding the steak and searing for about 3 minutes per side, until the steak is deep brown and crisp. Allow the meat to rest for 5 to 10 minutes before serving.

**Per Serving** Total Calories: 345; Total Fat: 23g; Saturated Fat: 7g; Cholesterol: 75mg; Sodium: 63mg; Potassium: 220mg; Total Carbohydrate: 8g; Fiber: 3g; Sugars: 1g; Protein: 26g

# BEEF-AND-BEAN CHILI

**30-MINUTE**
**ONE POT**

**PREP** 5 minutes
**COOK** 20 minutes

1 pound lean or extra-lean ground beef

1 yellow onion, diced

3 (15-ounce) cans no-salt diced tomatoes with green chilies (Ro-Tel brand)

2 (15-ounce) cans beans, drained and rinsed (whatever you desire: black, red, pinto, kidney, etc.)

2 tablespoons chili powder

*Optional:* 1 (10-ounce) package frozen spinach

*serves 4* **A classic comfort food, chili is a traditional dish often made of ground beef, chili powder, beans, and tomatoes. This recipe keeps it simple and delicious—it makes use of just a handful of ingredients and takes less than 30 minutes to prepare. For a chili that is more suited to the DASH diet, give the optional spinach a try. Freeze the leftovers so you have something healthy on hand when you don't feel like cooking.**

1. In a large stockpot, cook the beef over medium-high heat until browned, stirring frequently. Using a slotted spoon, transfer the cooked beef to a separate plate and set aside. Reserve 1 tablespoon of grease in the stockpot and discard the rest.

2. Add the onion to the stockpot and sauté for 4 to 5 minutes until soft.

3. Add the tomatoes with green chilies, beans, chili powder, and cooked beef to the stockpot, and stir to combine. Bring to a boil, reduce heat to medium-low. Cover and simmer for 10 minutes.

4. Serve immediately.

**BUDGET-SAVER TIP** If it fits your budget, choose lean or extra-lean ground beef. Regular ground beef has the highest fat content, about 25 to 30 percent, since it is cut from the trimmings of inexpensive cuts like brisket and shank. Too much saturated fat in the diet contributes to heart disease.

---

**Per Serving** Total Calories: 429; Total Fat: 10g; Saturated Fat: 3g; Cholesterol: 65mg; Sodium: 322mg; Potassium: 816mg; Total Carbohydrate: 47g; Fiber: 16g; Sugars: 0g; Protein: 38g

# GLAZED GRILLED PORK RIBS WITH HONEY, GINGER, AND SOY SAUCE

**PREP** 1 hour
**COOK** 30 minutes

4 pounds baby back ribs

1 tablespoon fresh ginger, grated

6 garlic cloves, finely chopped

1 teaspoon salt

2 teaspoons freshly ground black pepper

¼ cup honey

2 tablespoons low-sodium soy sauce

1 teaspoon olive oil

**SUBSTITUTION TIP** You can substitute half of the soy sauce with Asian fish sauce. Fish sauce will give the dish an umami flavor, the fifth taste element known for adding an incredible depth of flavor to practically any recipe. A little goes a long way, so start with a small amount and taste before adding more.

*serves 4* **This recipe should be viewed as a special-occasion treat, as pork ribs do not meet the USDA guidelines for lean cuts of meat. However, pork is a rich source of essential nutrients, vitamins, and minerals. When eaten in moderation and prepared in a low-fat manner, such as grilling, pork can play an important role in a healthy varied diet. A surprisingly good source of potassium, 1 serving of ribs provides 11 percent of your recommended daily intake.**

1. Place the ribs in a nonreactive baking dish just large enough to hold them in a single layer.

2. In a small bowl, whisk the ginger, garlic, salt, pepper, honey, and soy sauce together. Spread the glaze over the ribs on both sides. Let the ribs marinate in the refrigerator, covered, for 1 hour or more. The longer the ribs marinate the richer the flavor.

3. Prepare a grill for medium heat. Apply olive oil to the grill rack.

4. Place ribs, bone-side down, on the hot grate. Grill until golden brown and cooked through, about 8 to 12 minutes per side. When the ribs are done, the meat will have shrunk back from the bones by about ¼ inch.

5. Transfer the racks of ribs to a cutting board and cut them into individual ribs, then arrange them on a platter or on plates for serving.

**Per Serving** Total Calories: 805; Total Fat: 39g; Saturated Fat: 13g; Cholesterol: 290mg; Sodium: 620mg; Potassium: 1591mg; Total Carbohydrate: 21g; Fiber: 0g; Sugars: 19g; Protein: 88g

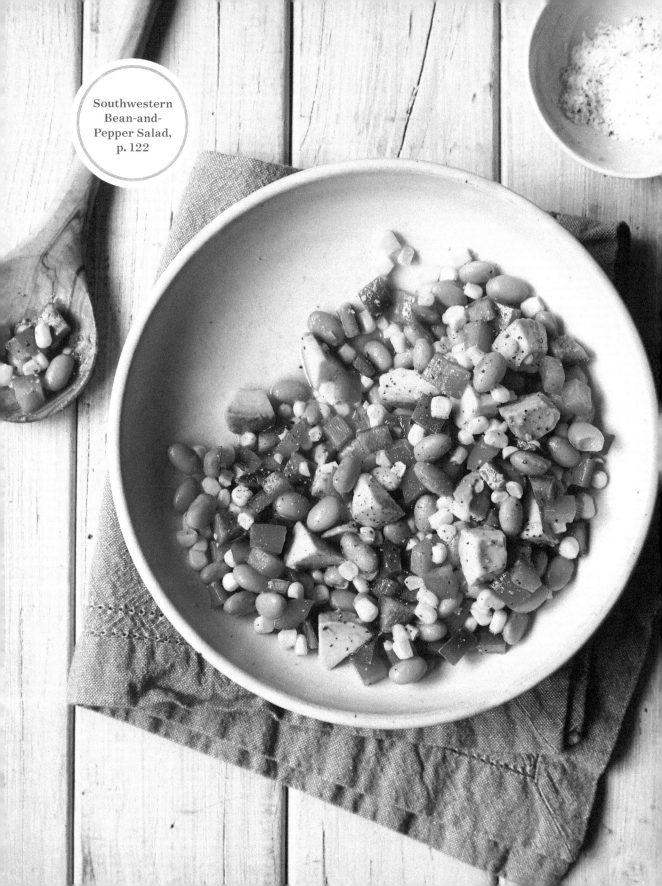

Southwestern
Bean-and-
Pepper Salad,
p. 122

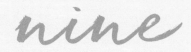
*nine*

# Snacks, Sides & Desserts

Southwestern Bean-
and-Pepper Salad  **122**

Cauliflower Mashed
"Potatoes"  **123**

Roasted Brussels
Sprouts  **124**

Broccoli with Garlic
and Lemon  **125**

Brown-Rice Pilaf  **126**

Chunky Black-Bean Dip  **127**

Classic Hummus  **128**

Crispy Potato Skins  **129**

Roasted Chickpeas  **130**

Carrot-Cake
Smoothie  **131**

Easy Cinnamon
Baked Apples  **132**

Chocolate Cake
in a Mug  **133**

Peanut Butter Banana
"Ice Cream"  **134**

Banana-Cashew
Cream Mousse  **135**

Peach and
Blueberry Tart  **136**

Sriracha Parsnip Fries  **137**

# SOUTHWESTERN BEAN-
# AND-PEPPER SALAD

VEGAN
30-MINUTE
BUDGET-SAVER

**PREP** 6 minutes

1 (15-ounce) can pinto
beans, drained and rinsed

2 bell peppers, cored
and chopped

1 cup corn kernels
(cut from 1 to 2 ears
or frozen and thawed)

Salt

Freshly ground black pepper

Juice of 2 limes

1 tablespoon olive oil

1 avocado, chopped

*serves 4* **This classic combination of colorful
salad ingredients makes a great side dish for grilled
meats and fish, topping for taco salads, or accom-
paniment to meat or vegetable fajitas. Loaded with
vitamins, minerals, and antioxidants, and with
protein from fiber-rich beans, this salad is a perfect
dish for a meatless dinner.**

1. In a large bowl, combine beans, peppers, corn, salt,
   and pepper. Squeeze fresh lime juice to taste and stir
   in olive oil. Let the mixture stand in the refrigerator for
   30 minutes.

2. Add avocado just before serving.

BUDGET-SAVER TIP Avocado prices can vary dramatically depending on their availability. And while avocado in your salad can really
add flavor and satiety, for an equally delicious salad you could add a
cup of cooked and chopped sweet potatoes with 1 to 2 tablespoons
of sunflower seeds.

---

**Per Serving** Total Calories: 245; Total Fat: 11g; Saturated
Fat: 2g; Cholesterol: 0mg; Sodium: 97mg; Potassium: 380mg;
Total Carbohydrate: 32g; Fiber: 10g; Sugars: 4g; Protein: 8g

# CAULIFLOWER MASHED "POTATOES"

**VEGAN**
**30-MINUTE**
**ONE POT**
**BUDGET-SAVER**

**PREP** 10 minutes
**COOK** 10 minutes

16 cups water (enough to cover cauliflower)

1 head cauliflower (about 3 pounds), trimmed and cut into florets

4 garlic cloves

1 tablespoon olive oil

¼ teaspoon salt

⅛ teaspoon freshly ground black pepper

2 teaspoons dried parsley

*serves 4* **One very easy way to add more vegetables to your diet is to replace some of your starchy carbs, like potatoes and pasta, with "mock" dishes created to be similar, but healthier and lower in calories. Mock mashed "potatoes" are made with cauliflower, a nutritional powerhouse with a similar silky texture to mashed potatoes. Serve this at your next Thanksgiving to really satisfy your guests.**

1. Bring a large pot of water to a boil. Add the cauliflower and garlic. Cook for about 10 minutes or until the cauliflower is fork tender. Drain, return it back to the hot pan, and let it stand for 2 to 3 minutes with the lid on.

2. Transfer the cauliflower and garlic to a food processor or blender. Add the olive oil, salt, and pepper, and purée until smooth.

3. Taste and adjust the salt and pepper. Remove to a serving bowl and add the parsley and mix until combined.

4. Garnish with additional olive oil, if desired. Serve immediately.

**INGREDIENT TIP** If you don't have a food processor or blender, you can make this dish just as you would traditional mashed potatoes by using a potato masher or hand blender.

**Per Serving** Total Calories: 87; Total Fat: 4g; Saturated Fat: 1g; Cholesterol: 0mg; Sodium: 210mg; Potassium: 654mg; Total Carbohydrate: 12g; Fiber: 5g; Sugars: 0g; Protein: 4g

# ROASTED BRUSSELS SPROUTS

VEGAN
30-MINUTE
SHEET PAN
BUDGET-SAVER

**PREP** 5 minutes
**COOK** 20 minutes

1½ pounds Brussels sprouts, trimmed and halved

2 tablespoons olive oil

¼ teaspoon salt

½ teaspoon freshly ground black pepper

*serves 4* Roasted Brussels sprouts are the perfect combination of savory and sweet. Brussels sprouts are a type of cruciferous vegetable (being a relative of the cabbage family) high in disease-protective nutrients. They are also a very good source of potassium and dietary fiber. This dish goes well with any meal, and the little cabbages are so delicious you might find they also make a terrific snack!

1. Preheat the oven to 400°F.

2. Combine the Brussels sprouts and olive oil in a large mixing bowl and toss until they are evenly coated.

3. Turn the Brussels sprouts out onto a large baking sheet and flip them over so they are cut-side down with the flat part touching the baking sheet. Sprinkle with salt and pepper.

4. Bake for 20 to 30 minutes or until the Brussels sprouts are lightly charred and crisp on the outside and toasted on the bottom. The outer leaves will be extra dark, too.

5. Serve immediately.

**INGREDIENT TIP** When choosing Brussels sprouts, look for bright-green heads that are firm and heavy for their size. The leaves should be tightly packed. Avoid sprouts with yellowing leaves—a sign of age—or black spots—which means they could have fungus.

**Per Serving** Total Calories: 134; Total Fat: 8g; Saturated Fat: 1g; Cholesterol: 0mg; Sodium: 189mg; Potassium: 665mg; Total Carbohydrate: 15g; Fiber: 7g; Sugars: 4g; Protein: 6g

# BROCCOLI WITH GARLIC AND LEMON

VEGAN
30-MINUTE
BUDGET-SAVER

**PREP** 2 minutes
**COOK** 4 minutes

1 cup water

4 cups broccoli florets

1 teaspoon olive oil

1 tablespoon minced garlic

1 teaspoon lemon zest

Salt

Freshly ground black pepper

*serves 4* **To fully reap the benefits of the DASH diet, be mindful of filling half of your plate at each meal with nutrient-dense, low-calorie vegetables. Filling up on vegetables not only helps with weight loss and weight management, but it adds those crucial blood-pressure-lowering nutrients to your diet. In this recipe, potassium- and magnesium-rich broccoli is brightly seasoned with lemon and garlic.**

1. In a small saucepan, bring 1 cup of water to a boil. Add the broccoli to the boiling water and cook for 2 to 3 minutes or until tender, being careful not to overcook. The broccoli should retain its bright-green color. Drain the water from the broccoli.

2. In a small sauté pan over medium-high heat, add the olive oil. Add the garlic and sauté for 30 seconds. Add the broccoli, lemon zest, salt, and pepper. Combine well and serve.

**INGREDIENT TIP** To retain the most nutrients in your vegetables, it is important not to overcook them, as the vitamins and minerals will leach out into the cooking water. Steamer baskets are inexpensive and are a good way to quickly cook veggies. Another method to minimize nutrient loss is to steam in the microwave by adding the vegetables to a microwave-safe dish with a couple of tablespoons of water and cooking on high for 2 to 3 minutes.

**Per Serving** Total Calories: 38; Total Fat: 1g; Saturated Fat: 0g; Cholesterol: 0mg; Sodium: 24mg; Potassium: 295mg; Total Carbohydrate: 5g; Fiber: 3g; Sugars: 0g; Protein: 3g

# BROWN-RICE PILAF

VEGAN
30-MINUTE
ONE POT
BUDGET-SAVER

**PREP** 5 minutes
**COOK** 10 minutes

1 cup low-sodium vegetable broth

½ tablespoon olive oil

1 clove garlic, minced

1 scallion, thinly sliced

1 tablespoon minced onion flakes

1 cup instant brown rice

⅛ teaspoon freshly ground black pepper

*serves 4* **The DASH diet recommends a slightly higher intake of whole grains than the Dietary Guidelines for Americans. Whole grains like brown rice are an excellent source of B vitamins, complex carbohydrates, and the mineral magnesium. Made with pantry staples in just 10 minutes, this rice pilaf is quick, simple, tasty, and healthy.**

1. Mix the vegetable broth, olive oil, garlic, scallion, and minced onion flakes in a saucepan and bring to a boil.

2. Add rice, return mixture to boil, then reduce heat and simmer for 10 minutes.

3. Remove from heat and let stand for 5 minutes.

4. Fluff with a fork and season with black pepper.

**INGREDIENT TIP** The nutritional differences between a serving of long-grain brown rice, which requires 35 to 45 minutes to cook, and instant brown rice, which cooks in about 10 minutes, is insignificant. Instant rice has simply been cooked and dehydrated so it cooks quicker than long-grain rice. Feel free to use both varieties interchangeably.

---

**Per Serving** Total Calories: 100; Total Fat: 2g; Saturated Fat: 0g; Cholesterol: 0mg; Sodium: 35mg; Potassium: 24mg; Total Carbohydrate: 19g; Fiber: 2g; Sugars: 1g; Protein: 2g

# CHUNKY BLACK-BEAN DIP

VEGETARIAN
30-MINUTE
BUDGET-SAVER

**YIELD** 2 cups
**PREP** 5 minutes

1 (15-ounce) can black beans, drained, with liquid reserved

½ (7-ounce) can chipotle peppers in adobo sauce

¼ cup plain Greek yogurt

Freshly ground black pepper

*serves 6–8* This black-bean dip makes a healthy snack and can help you increase your intake of beans and dairy, two DASH-recommended foods. Made with just three main ingredients, this dip is full of flavor and goes great paired with raw vegetables, mixed into hot grains, or used as a sandwich spread.

1. Combine beans, peppers, and yogurt in a food processor or blender and process until smooth. Add some of the bean liquid, 1 tablespoon at a time, for a thinner consistency.

2. Season to taste with black pepper.

3. Serve.

**INGREDIENT TIP** Chipotles are small peppers that have been dried by a smoking process that gives them a dark color and a distinct smoky flavor. You can find this canned ingredient in the Latin aisle of grocery stores and big-box chains. As an alternative, you could use 1 teaspoon dry chipotle chili powder.

**Per ⅓-Cup Serving** Total Calories: 70; Total Fat: 1g; Saturated Fat: 0g; Cholesterol: 0mg; Sodium: 159mg; Potassium: 21mg; Total Carbohydrate: 11g; Fiber: 4g; Sugars: 0g; Protein: 5g

# CLASSIC HUMMUS

VEGAN
30-MINUTE
ONE POT
BUDGET-SAVER

YIELD 2 cups
PREP 5 minutes

1 (15-ounce) can chickpeas, drained and rinsed

3 tablespoons sesame tahini

2 tablespoons olive oil

3 garlic cloves, chopped

Juice of 1 lemon

Salt

Freshly ground black pepper

*serves 6–8* Hummus is a creamy, thick spread made primarily from puréed chickpeas plus a few other healthy ingredients. Commonly consumed with every single meal in Israel, it is a large part of a Mediterranean diet, which has similar benefits to DASH and can reduce inflammation in the body. Making your own homemade hummus is extremely easy, takes just a few minutes, and costs pennies. Eat hummus with vegetable sticks or with whole-grain pita bread for a snack, or use it as a topping for salads.

1. In a food processor or blender, combine all the ingredients until smooth but thick. Add water if necessary to produce a smoother hummus.

2. Store covered for up to 5 days.

**INGREDIENT TIP** Supermarkets offer a variety of different flavors of hummus, which you can easily recreate at home. For red pepper hummus, simply add 1 chopped red pepper to the ingredients. Try beets, cucumber, olives, or avocado. The possibilities are endless.

---

**Per ⅓-Cup Serving** Total Calories: 147; Total Fat: 10g; Saturated Fat: 1g; Cholesterol: 0mg; Sodium: 64mg; Potassium: 16mg; Total Carbohydrate: 11g; Fiber: 4g; Sugars: 0g; Protein: 6g

# CRISPY POTATO SKINS

VEGAN
30-MINUTE
ONE POT
BUDGET-SAVER

**PREP** 2 minutes
**COOK** 19 minutes

2 russet potatoes

Cooking spray

1 teaspoon dried rosemary

⅛ teaspoon freshly ground black pepper

**INGREDIENT TIP** You can use any type of potato in this recipe: Yukon gold, red, or sweet. Whatever fits your budget. You could also boost the calcium in this recipe by sprinkling shredded cheese on the skins before baking.

*serves 2* **Russet potatoes are a good source of several DASH-recommended minerals, including magnesium and calcium. They are also very nutritious, as long as you watch portion sizes. This quick and tasty recipe makes it easy to enjoy potatoes, as it uses just their skins, which are the most nutritious and fiber-rich parts of the potato. Adapt this recipe to your personal tastes by varying the seasonings.**

1. Preheat the oven to 375°F.

2. Wash the potatoes and pierce several times with a fork. Place on a plate. Cook on full power in the microwave for 5 minutes. Turn over, and continue to cook for 3 to 4 minutes more, or until soft.

3. Carefully—the potatoes will be very hot—cut the potatoes in half and scoop out the pulp, leaving about ⅛ inch of potato flesh attached to the skin. Save the pulp for another use.

4. Spray the inside of each potato with cooking spray. Press in the rosemary and pepper. Place the skins on a baking sheet and bake in preheated oven for 5 to 10 minutes until slightly browned and crispy.

5. Serve immediately.

**Per Serving** Total Calories: 114; Total Fat: 0g; Saturated Fat: 0g; Cholesterol: 0mg; Sodium: 0mg; Potassium: 635mg; Total Carbohydrate: 27g; Fiber: 2g; Sugars: 1g; Protein: 3g

# ROASTED CHICKPEAS

**VEGAN**
**ONE POT**
**BUDGET-SAVER**

**PREP** 5 minutes
**COOK** 30 minutes

1 (15-ounce can) chickpeas, drained and rinsed

½ teaspoon olive oil

2 teaspoons of your favorite herbs or spice blend

¼ teaspoon salt

*serves 2* **Following a healthy diet doesn't mean you have to give up crunchy, tasty snacks. Remember, you always want to think of how you can *add* nutrients to your diet. So with that principle in mind, this simple roasted-chickpeas recipe uses a handful of pantry ingredients to create a delicious, nutritious, crunchy, positively addictive snack that you can feel good about eating.**

1. Preheat the oven to 400°F.

2. Drain and rinse the chickpeas. Spread a layer of paper towels on a rimmed baking sheet and spread the chickpeas on top. Blot the top with more paper towels until the chickpeas are relatively dry.

3. Place the dried chickpeas in a medium bowl. Drizzle in the olive oil and toss gently with a large spoon. Sprinkle on the herbs and salt and toss again.

4. Spread chickpeas on the baking sheet in a single layer.

5. Bake for 30 to 40 minutes, stirring halfway through, until golden brown and crunchy.

6. Serve.

**INGREDIENT TIP** If you like everything bagels, try mixing together 1 teaspoon each: sesame seeds, poppy seeds, dried minced onion, and dried minced garlic—use this mixture as the seasoning in this recipe to make everything roasted chickpeas.

---

**Per Serving** Total Calories: 175; Total Fat: 3g; Saturated Fat: 0g; Cholesterol: 0mg; Sodium: 474mg; Potassium: 0mg; Total Carbohydrate: 29g; Fiber: 11g; Sugars: 0g; Protein: 11g

# CARROT-CAKE SMOOTHIE

VEGETARIAN
30-MINUTE
BUDGET-SAVER

**PREP** 5 minutes

1 frozen banana, peeled
and diced

1 cup carrots, diced
(peeled if preferred)

1 cup nonfat or low-fat milk

½ cup nonfat or low-fat
vanilla Greek yogurt

½ cup ice

¼ cup diced pineapple, frozen

½ teaspoon ground cinnamon

Pinch nutmeg

*Optional toppings:* chopped
walnuts, grated carrots

*serves 2* **Enjoy a classic dessert favorite in the form of a healthier smoothie. This nutritious carrot-cake smoothie is made with antioxidant- and potassium-rich carrots, calcium, and protein-rich Greek yogurt, and has all of the taste of traditional carrot cake with the addition of pineapple, walnuts, and carrot-cake spices.**

1. Add all of the ingredients to a blender and process until smooth and creamy.

2. Serve immediately with optional toppings as desired.

**INGREDIENT TIP** You could also use plain Greek yogurt or plain regular yogurt and add your own sweetener to this recipe. Good choices are 1 to 2 teaspoons of pure maple syrup or honey. You could also opt for a no-calorie sweetener like stevia.

**Per Serving** Total Calories: 180; Total Fat: 1g; Saturated Fat: 0g; Cholesterol: 5mg; Sodium: 114mg; Potassium: 682mg; Total Carbohydrate: 36g; Fiber: 4g; Sugars: 25g; Protein: 10g

# EASY CINNAMON BAKED APPLES

VEGAN
BUDGET-SAVER

**PREP** 5 minutes
**COOK** 45 minutes

4 apples, cored, peeled, and sliced thin

½ tablespoon ground cinnamon

¼ cup brown sugar

¼ teaspoon ground nutmeg

*Optional:* 2 teaspoons freshly squeezed lemon juice

*serves 4* **This simple recipe for cinnamon baked apples tastes like a cobbler or pie without the crust. While most recipes for baked apples bake the entire apple, this variation uses apple slices. Satisfying and sweet, this recipe makes a perfect dessert or breakfast with Greek yogurt.**

1. Preheat the oven to 375°F.

2. Place apples in a mixing bowl and gently mix all the other ingredients together.

3. Put apples in a nonstick pan. Cover and place in the oven.

4. Bake for 45 minutes, stirring at least once every 15 minutes. Once they are soft, cook for another few minutes to thicken the cinnamon sauce.

5. Serve.

**INGREDIENT TIP** Choose your favorite variety of apple or the type that fits your budget. Rome Beauty is a type that is perfectly suited for baking, but any variety works well in this recipe.

---

**Per Serving** Total Calories: 117; Total Fat: 1g; Saturated Fat: 0g; Cholesterol: 0mg; Sodium: 4mg; Potassium: 206mg; Total Carbohydrate: 34g; Fiber: 5g; Sugars: 28g; Protein: 0g

# CHOCOLATE CAKE IN A MUG

**VEGETARIAN**
**30-MINUTE**
**BUDGET-SAVER**

**PREP** 5 minutes
**COOK** 1 minute

3 tablespoons white whole-wheat flour

2 tablespoons unsweetened cocoa powder

2 teaspoons sugar

⅛ teaspoon baking powder

1 egg white

½ teaspoon olive oil

3 tablespoons nonfat or low-fat milk

½ teaspoon vanilla extract

Cooking spray

*serves 1* When a chocolate craving hits, satisfy it in minutes with this sinfully delicious, yet very nutritious, chocolate cake in a mug. Cocoa is an excellent source of flavonoids, a type of plant chemical with disease-protective qualities. Cocoa may also lower bad LDL cholesterol and improve blood pressure due to its high amounts of calcium and potassium. Now you have a justifiable and healthy reason to include cocoa regularly in your diet.

1. Place the flour, cocoa, sugar, and baking powder in a small bowl and whisk until combined. Then add in the egg white, olive oil, milk, and vanilla extract, and mix to combine.

2. Spray a mug with cooking spray and pour batter into mug. Microwave on high for 60 seconds or until set.

3. Serve.

**INGREDIENT TIP** Choose a whole-grain flour for the most nutrients, including B vitamins, minerals, and fiber. Other good choices include whole-wheat pastry flour, spelt flour, and kamut flour.

**Per Serving** Total Calories: 217; Total Fat: 4g; Saturated Fat: 1g; Cholesterol: 1mg; Sodium: 139mg; Potassium: 244mg; Total Carbohydrate: 35g; Fiber: 7g; Sugars: 12g; Protein: 11g

# PEANUT BUTTER BANANA "ICE CREAM"

**VEGAN**
**30-MINUTE**
**BUDGET-SAVER**

**PREP** 10 minutes

4 bananas, very ripe

2 tablespoons peanut butter

*serves 4* **You may be skeptical about this recipe, which uses just two ingredients to create ice cream without cream, milk, butter, eggs, or sugar. This recipe results in a smooth and creamy texture that is so similar to ice cream.**

1. Peel bananas and slice into ½-inch disks. Arrange banana slices on a large plate or baking sheet. Freeze for 1 to 2 hours.

2. Place the banana slices in a food processor or powerful blender. Purée banana slices, scraping down the bowl as needed. Purée until the mixture is creamy and smooth. Add the peanut butter and purée to combine. Serve immediately for soft-serve ice cream consistency. If you prefer harder ice cream, place in the freezer for a few hours, then serve.

**INGREDIENT TIP** If you have a hard time creating a creamy consistency, you can add 1 to 2 tablespoons of milk to help purée the banana slices.

**Per Serving** Total Calories: 153; Total Fat: 4g; Saturated Fat: 1g; Cholesterol: 0mg; Sodium: 4mg; Potassium: 422mg; Total Carbohydrate: 29g; Fiber: 4g; Sugars: 15g; Protein: 3g

# BANANA-CASHEW CREAM MOUSSE

**PREP** 55 minutes, plus 2 to 3 hours for soaking cashews

½ cup cashews, presoaked

1 tablespoon honey

1 teaspoon vanilla extract

1 large banana, sliced (reserve 4 slices for garnish)

1 cup plain nonfat Greek yogurt

*serves 2* This quick banana-cashew cream mousse recipe makes and unbelievably satisfying and heart-healthy snack or dessert. Perfectly suited to the DASH eating plan, each serving contains ample amounts of calcium, magnesium, potassium, healthy fats, and protein. It can help you meet your goals for several food groups including dairy, nuts, and protein. Light and fluffy with a creamy texture, you can even eat this for breakfast.

1. Place the cashews in a small bowl and cover with 1 cup of water. Soak at room temperature for 2 to 3 hours. Drain, rinse, and set aside.

2. Place honey, vanilla extract, cashews, and bananas in a blender or food processor. Blend until smooth.

3. Place mixture in a medium bowl. Fold in yogurt, mix well. Cover.

4. Chill in refrigerator, covered, for at least 45 minutes.

5. Portion mousse into 2 serving bowls. Garnish each with 2 banana slices.

**INGREDIENT TIP** Soaking nuts is thought to remove their enzyme inhibitors and reduce their phytic acid content, making them easier to digest and their nutrients more easily absorbed. Soaking may also remove potential irritants such as mold and pesticides.

**Per Serving** Total Calories: 329; Total Fat: 14g; Saturated Fat: 3g; Cholesterol: 8mg; Sodium: 64mg; Potassium: 507mg; Total Carbohydrate: 37g; Fiber: 3g; Sugars: 24g; Protein: 17g

# PEACH AND BLUEBERRY TART

VEGETARIAN

**PREP** 10 minutes
**COOK** 30 minutes

1 sheet frozen puff pastry

1 cup fresh blueberries

4 peaches, pitted and sliced

3 tablespoons sugar

2 tablespoons cornstarch

1 tablespoon freshly squeezed lemon juice

Cooking spray

1 tablespoon nonfat or low-fat milk

Confectioners' sugar, for dusting

**SUBSTITUTION TIP** You could substitute the pastry puff with a premade graham-cracker or shortbread crust, or you can make your own crust. You could also use mini tart shells for better portion control.

*serves 6–8* This fruit tart is a foolproof dessert that you can count on to be a crowd-pleaser. Keep frozen puff pastry on hand, or see the tip below for more ideas. This is a great recipe to make during peak blueberry and peach season, and it can be made in a snap. With a larger yield than the other recipes in this book, this dessert is perfect when you want leftovers or need a dish to share.

1. Thaw puff pastry at room temperature for at least 30 minutes.

2. Preheat the oven to 400°F.

3. In a large bowl, toss the blueberries, peaches, sugar, cornstarch, and lemon juice.

4. Spray a round pie pan with cooking spray.

5. Unfold pastry and place on prepared pie pan.

6. Arrange the peach slices so they are slightly overlapping. Spread the blueberries on top of the peaches.

7. Drape pastry over the outside of the fruit and press pleats firmly together. Brush with milk.

8. Bake in the bottom third of the oven until crust is golden, about 30 minutes.

9. Cool on a rack.

10. Sprinkle pastry with confectioners' sugar. Serve.

**Per Serving** Total Calories: 119; Total Fat: 3g; Saturated Fat: 1g; Cholesterol: 0mg; Sodium: 21mg; Potassium: 155mg; Total Carbohydrate: 23g; Fiber: 2g; Sugars: 15g; Protein: 1g

# SRIRACHA PARSNIP FRIES

**VEGETARIAN**
**BUDGET-SAVER**
**SHEET PAN**

**PREP** 10 minutes
**COOK** 25 minutes

1 pound parsnips, peeled, cut into 3 × ½-inch strips

1 tablespoon olive oil

1 teaspoon dried rosemary

Sriracha to taste

Salt and pepper to taste

**INGREDIENT TIP** Choose firm, medium parsnips because larger ones are more fibrous and difficult to cook. Avoid those with lots of whiskers and brown patches because these generally indicate a poor-quality harvest.

*serves 4* Parsnips are one of those vegetables that are not often given the attention they deserve for their many healthy benefits. Resembling a carrot but white in color, parsnips can help maintain a healthy heart and blood pressure. A 1-cup serving of parsnips contains a whopping 499 milligrams of potassium, 7 grams of cholesterol-lowering fiber, and high levels of folate, which can help to relax blood vessels. This parsnip fries recipe is so good you may never eat French fries again.

1. Preheat oven to 450°F.

2. Mix parsnips, rosemary, and oil in a medium size bowl. Season with salt, pepper, and sriracha to taste and toss to coat.

3. Lay parsnips on a baking sheet making sure the strips don't overlap. (If they are touching they will become mushy instead of crispy.)

4. Bake for 10 minutes. Turn and roast until parsnips are browned in spots, 10 to 15 minutes longer. If you want them to be extra crispy, turn the broiler on for the last 2 to 3 minutes.

5. Remove from oven and enjoy.

**Per Serving** Total Calories: 112; Total Fat: 4g; Saturated Fat: 1g; Cholesterol: 0mg; Sodium: 12mg; Potassium: 419mg; Total Carbohydrate: 20g; Fiber: 4g; Sugars: 5g; Protein: 2g

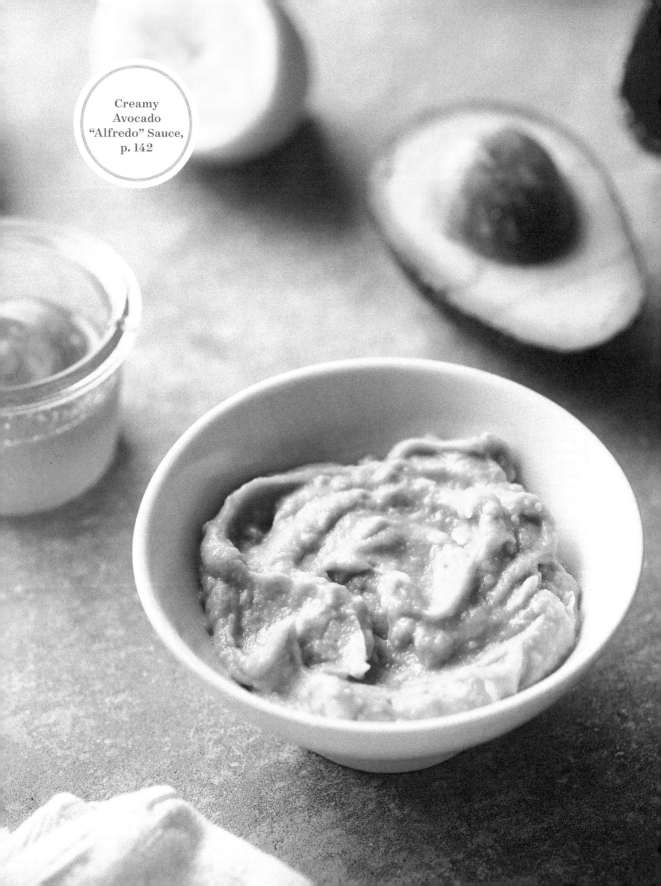

Creamy
Avocado
"Alfredo" Sauce,
p. 142

*ten*

# Broths, Condiments & Sauces

Super Simple
Vegetable Broth 140

Quick Chicken Stock 141

Creamy Avocado
"Alfredo" Sauce 142

Tomato-Basil Sauce 143

Red Pepper Pesto 144

Cranberry Sauce 145

Greek Yogurt
Mayonnaise 146

Fresh Vegetable Salsa 147

Tangy Barbecue Sauce 148

Spiced Pepper Relish 149

# SUPER SIMPLE VEGETABLE BROTH

**VEGAN**
**ONE POT**

**PREP** 5 minutes
**COOK** 1 hour 30 minutes

4 carrots, peeled

1 large onion, peeled

3 celery stalks

1 leek, trimmed and thoroughly washed

2 small potatoes, scrubbed but not peeled

2 garlic cloves, peeled

2 teaspoons dried thyme

½ tablespoon dried parsley

1 bay leaf

1 teaspoon salt

1 teaspoon whole peppercorns

8 cups water

*makes 4–6 cups* **Making your own vegetable broth is very easy to do. It's inexpensive and much healthier than processed varieties. This simple broth can be eaten as is or used as a base for soups and chili recipes. Adapt the recipe to the vegetables you have on hand.**

1. Chop carrots, onion, celery, and leek into 1- to 2-inch chunks. Leave the potatoes whole. Combine the vegetables with the remaining ingredients in a soup pot or stockpot. Add water and bring to a boil. Reduce heat to maintain a simmer for 1 hour.

2. Strain the broth through a colander, then once more through a fine sieve. If the broth tastes weak, pour it back into the pot and simmer until reduced to a flavor you prefer, 20 to 30 minutes more.

**SUBSTITUTION TIP** You can make substitutions with the vegetables depending on their cost and availability. Instead of a leek, you could use 2 onions, or try adding a turnip instead.

**Per 1-Cup Serving** Total Calories: 100; Total Fat: 0g; Saturated Fat: 0g; Cholesterol: 0mg; Sodium: 544mg; Potassium: 633mg; Total Carbohydrate: 24g; Fiber: 4g; Sugars: 4g; Protein: 3g

# QUICK CHICKEN STOCK

**ONE POT**

**PREP** 15 minutes
**COOK** 30 minutes

4 pounds chicken carcasses, including necks and backs

½ large onion, roughly chopped

2 large carrots, roughly chopped

1 celery stalk, roughly chopped

1 bay leaf

3 garlic cloves

4 cups water

*makes 3 cups* **Making your own chicken stock is inexpensive, is easy to throw together—and needs no more than just a few basic ingredients. When making your own stock, you know the ingredients are fresh and you can control the amount of added salt, important for keeping your blood pressure in check. You can also freeze homemade stock, so you have it on hand to use in other recipes.**

1. Combine the chicken carcasses with onion, carrots, celery, bay leaf, and garlic in a large pot with 4 cups of water, and turn the heat to high.

2. Bring almost to a boil, then lower the heat so the mixture sends up a few bubbles at a time. Cook for 30 to 60 minutes.

3. Cool slightly and strain, pressing down on the solids in the strainer to extract as much liquid as possible. Discard the solids.

**BUDGET-SAVER TIP**  This recipe is a good use for leftover rotisserie chicken and can help you reduce food waste.

**Per 1-Cup Serving**  Total Calories: 208; Total Fat: 6g; Saturated Fat: 1g; Cholesterol: 109mg; Sodium: 196mg; Potassium: 609mg; Total Carbohydrate: 9g; Fiber: 2g; Sugars: 2g; Protein: 29g

# CREAMY AVOCADO "ALFREDO" SAUCE

**VEGAN**
**30-MINUTE**
**BUDGET-SAVER**

**PREP**  10 minutes

1 ripe avocado, peeled and pitted

1 tablespoon dried basil

1 clove garlic

1 tablespoon lemon juice

1 tablespoon olive oil

⅛ teaspoon salt

*serves 4*  **This lightened-up version of Alfredo sauce uses creamy, fiber-rich avocado in place of heavy cream. It can be served warm or cold and can be made in advance and stored in the refrigerator. Made in a blender, this sauce sticks well to pasta noodles or vegetable noodles. The best part is that the entire recipe costs just a couple of dollars to make.**

1. Add the avocado, basil, garlic clove, lemon juice, olive oil, and salt to a food processor. Blend until a smooth, creamy sauce forms.

2. Pour the sauce over hot pasta or vegetable noodles.

**INGREDIENT TIP**  Avocados oxidize and turn brown quickly once cut, so if you plan on making this in advance, cover it with a thin layer of lemon or lime juice before refrigerating in a container. When ready to use, pour the juice off or stir it in.

---

**Per Serving**  Total Calories: 104; Total Fat: 10g; Saturated Fat: 1g; Cholesterol: 0mg; Sodium: 43mg; Potassium: 229mg; Total Carbohydrate: 4g; Fiber: 3g; Sugars: 0g; Protein: 1g

# TOMATO-BASIL SAUCE

**VEGAN**
**30-MINUTE**
**ONE POT**
**BUDGET-SAVER**

**PREP** 5 minutes
**COOK** 10 minutes

2 tablespoons olive oil

3 garlic cloves, finely chopped

4 (15-ounce) cans no-salt, crushed, or chopped tomatoes

1 tablespoon dried basil

Salt

Freshly ground black pepper

*serves 6* **This quick and easy tomato-basil sauce goes well with pasta, meat, fish, beans, and vegetables. Made with pantry staples, the sauce is a great source of blood-pressure-lowering potassium as well as the antioxidant vitamin C. For even more nutrition, consider adding 1 to 2 cups of your favorite vegetables.**

1. Heat the oil in a large saucepan and sauté the garlic for about a minute until lightly browned, being careful not to burn. Add the tomatoes and basil, season with salt and pepper, and cook uncovered over medium heat for about 10 minutes.

2. Serve over pasta, grains, beans, or vegetables.

**SUBSTITUTION TIP** When fresh tomatoes are in season, replace each can of tomatoes with 2 cups of chopped fresh tomatoes and their juices. Though you could use any type of tomato, tomatoes like Roma—used for making tomato paste due to their meaty texture and little to no seeds—are said to develop the best flavor when cooked down to a sauce.

**Per Serving** Total Calories: 103; Total Fat: 5g; Saturated Fat: 1g; Cholesterol: 0mg; Sodium: 32mg; Potassium: 735mg; Total Carbohydrate: 15g; Fiber: 3g; Sugars: 0g; Protein: 3g

# RED PEPPER PESTO

**VEGETARIAN**
**30-MINUTE**

**PREP**  20 minutes
**COOK**  10 minutes

4 red bell peppers, tops sliced off and deseeded

3 cups fresh basil leaves

3 tablespoons cashews

3 tablespoons grated Parmesan cheese

1 tablespoon olive oil

3 garlic cloves

¼ teaspoon salt

*makes 3 cups* Red bell peppers are an excellent source of inflammation-reducing carotenoids, the antioxidant vitamin C, and a good source of the blood-pressure-lowering minerals potassium and magnesium. Used in this simple and nutritious recipe for pesto, the red peppers are first roasted in the oven for added flavor and sweetness. Serve the pesto as a dip for bread, over whole-grain pasta, or mixed into steamed vegetables.

1. Place peppers in the oven on a sheet pan and turn broiler to high. Broil until peppers have blackened on all sides, turning a few times, for about 10 minutes total.

2. Remove peppers from heat and place in a bowl. Cover with plastic wrap and set aside to cool.

3. Peel the cooled peppers. In a food processor, combine peeled peppers with the remaining ingredients. Process until mixture is smooth and resembles a pesto.

**SUBSTITUTION TIP**  Traditional pesto is made with pine nuts, which you can substitute for the cashews. To be more economical, you could also substitute sunflower seeds, or even for pumpkin seeds.

**Per ¼-Cup Serving**  Total Calories: 50; Total Fat: 3g; Saturated Fat: 0g; Cholesterol: 1mg; Sodium: 74mg; Potassium: 185mg; Total Carbohydrate: 5g; Fiber: 1g; Sugars: 0g; Protein: 2g

# CRANBERRY SAUCE

**VEGAN**
**ONE POT**
**BUDGET-SAVER**

**PREP** 5 minutes
**COOK** 10 minutes, plus
30 minutes cooling time

½ cup sugar

½ cup water

1 (12-ounce) package fresh
or frozen cranberries

½ teaspoon ground cinnamon

*Optional:* 2 tablespoons 100%
orange juice

*makes 2¼ cups* **Cranberries have an amazing array of phytonutrients that offer cardio-vascular and immune support, protection against urinary-tract infections, and anti-inflammatory benefits. One of the most nutrient-rich berries out there, cranberries are inexpensive and are available year round, fresh or frozen. This simple recipe uses just a couple of ingredients. Serve this delicious sauce as a side to cooked fish or meat.**

1. Combine all the ingredients in a medium saucepan. Bring to a boil over medium-high heat, then reduce to a simmer. Cook, stirring occasionally, until berries start to pop. Press berries against side of the pan with a wooden spoon and continue to cook, until berries are completely broken down and achieve a jam-like consistency, about 10 minutes total.

2. Remove from heat and allow to cool for about 30 minutes. Stir in water in 1-tablespoon increments to adjust to desired consistency.

3. Serve immediately or store in the refrigerator for 10 to 14 days. You can also freeze the sauce and, for best results, aim to use it within 1 to 2 months.

**BUDGET-SAVER TIP** Buy several bags of cranberries when they are in season and on sale. Store them in the freezer without opening or washing. When ready to use, simply wash and drain.

**Per ¼ Cup Serving** Total Calories: 113; Total Fat: 0g; Saturated Fat: 0g; Cholesterol: 0mg; Sodium: 0mg; Potassium: 1mg; Total Carbohydrate: 29g; Fiber: 3g; Sugars: 26g; Protein: 0g

# GREEK YOGURT MAYONNAISE

**VEGETARIAN**
**30-MINUTE**
**BUDGET-SAVER**

**PREP** 2 minutes

6 ounces nonfat or low-fat plain Greek yogurt

1 teaspoon apple cider vinegar

¼ teaspoon yellow mustard

¼ teaspoon hot sauce

¼ teaspoon freshly ground black pepper

¼ teaspoon paprika

¼ teaspoon salt

*serves 12* Mayonnaise is not known as a healthy condiment, even though it is a staple in many homes. You can make a much healthier spread that's high in DASH-recommended nutrients in just a few minutes. Greek yogurt has a similar thick consistency and works as a great base for a homemade version. Greek yogurt is also high in calcium and is packed with protein (keeping you feeling full) and probiotics that aid in digestion. Adjust the spices to suit your tastes.

Mix all the ingredients together and blend well. Adjust seasonings to suit taste.

**INGREDIENT TIP** Greek yogurt is a staple you might consider keeping on hand when following the DASH diet. Try it as an alternative for heavy cream, add a pinch of salt and use in place of sour cream, add spices and a bit of milk for a creamy salad dressing, or simply enjoy plain as a snack.

**Per 2-Tablespoon Serving** Total Calories: 8; Total Fat: 0g; Saturated Fat: 0g; Cholesterol: 0mg; Sodium: 65mg; Potassium: 2mg; Total Carbohydrate: 1g; Fiber: 0g; Sugars: 1g; Protein: 1g

# FRESH VEGETABLE SALSA

**VEGETARIAN**
**30-MINUTE**
**ONE POT**

**PREP** 10 minutes

2 cups cored and diced
bell peppers

2 cups diced tomatoes

1 cup diced zucchini

½ cup chopped red onion

¼ cup freshly squeezed
lime juice

2 garlic cloves, minced

1 teaspoon freshly ground
black pepper

¼ teaspoon salt

*makes 6 cups* Store-bought salsa is surprisingly high in sodium and, while the DASH diet doesn't restrict sodium, too much of this mineral can contribute to high blood pressure. Making your own fresh salsa is easy, and this recipe uses a mix of vegetables high in potassium and magnesium, keeping added salt in check. Adapt this recipe to your personal preferences for heat and types of vegetables.

1. Wash the vegetables and prepare as directed.

2. In a large bowl, combine all the ingredients. Toss gently to mix.

3. Cover and refrigerate for at least 30 minutes to allow the flavors to blend.

**SUBSTITUTION TIP** If you prefer hotter salsa, add ½ to 1 tablespoon of finely chopped, seeded jalapeño peppers. You could also make this a bean salsa by adding ½ cup of black or pinto beans.

**Per ¼-Cup Serving** Total Calories: 10; Total Fat: 0g; Saturated Fat: 0g; Cholesterol: 0mg; Sodium: 26mg; Potassium: 81mg; Total Carbohydrate: 2g; Fiber: 1g; Sugars: 1g; Protein: 0g

# TANGY BARBECUE SAUCE

VEGETARIAN
30-MINUTE
BUDGET-SAVER

**PREP** 5 minutes

1 (8-ounce) can no-salt tomato paste

2 tablespoons Dijon mustard

1½ tablespoons apple cider vinegar

1 tablespoon low-sodium soy sauce

2 teaspoons molasses

1 teaspoon garlic powder

1 teaspoon onion powder

*makes 1½ cups* Most brands of barbecue sauce contain quite a bit of sugar, sodium, and preservatives. In fact, many recipes for homemade sauce use bottled ketchup as one of the main ingredients. This recipe is lower in sodium and takes just minutes to prepare.

1. In a medium bowl, whisk together all the ingredients until thoroughly combined.

2. Store in an airtight container in the refrigerator for up to a week.

**SUBSTITUTION TIP** You can adapt this recipe to your personal barbecue-sauce preferences and make it sweeter or give it extra spice. For more kick, add 1 teaspoon of chili powder, and for a sweeter flavor, add 1 to 2 packets of no-calorie sweetener. You could also make this a honey sauce by swapping molasses for honey.

**Per ¼-Cup Serving** Total Calories: 32; Total Fat: 0g; Saturated Fat: 0g; Cholesterol: 0mg; Sodium: 240mg; Potassium: 340mg; Total Carbohydrate: 7g; Fiber: 1g; Sugars: 4g; Protein: 2g

# SPICED PEPPER RELISH

VEGAN
ONE POT
BUDGET-SAVER

**PREP** 5 minutes
**COOK** 35 minutes

4 red bell peppers, cored and shredded

2 large onions, shredded

1 cup sugar

1 cup white wine vinegar

½ cup water

½ teaspoon salt

1 teaspoon crushed red pepper

*makes 5 cups* Adding vegetable relish to sandwiches or salads, or spooning it over beans, are great ways to sneak more vegetables into your diet, without even noticing it. Homemade relish is very easy to make, is inexpensive, and can be stored in the refrigerator for up to a month. This relish recipe is similar to traditional sweet-pickle relish but with a peppery kick.

1. Combine all the ingredients in a large saucepan; bring to a boil. Reduce heat, and simmer, uncovered, for 35 minutes or until thick, stirring frequently.

2. Cool, pour into airtight containers, and store in the refrigerator for up to 1 month.

**INGREDIENT TIP** Relish can be mixed into Greek yogurt to make a dip, puréed into a salad dressing, served on burgers, and mixed into ground meats. Get creative in the ways you boost your daily intake of vegetables.

**Per 2-Tablespoon Serving** Total Calories: 28; Total Fat: 0g; Saturated Fat: 0g; Cholesterol: 0mg; Sodium: 30mg; Potassium: 52mg; Total Carbohydrate: 7g; Fiber: 0g; Sugars: 5g; Protein: 0g

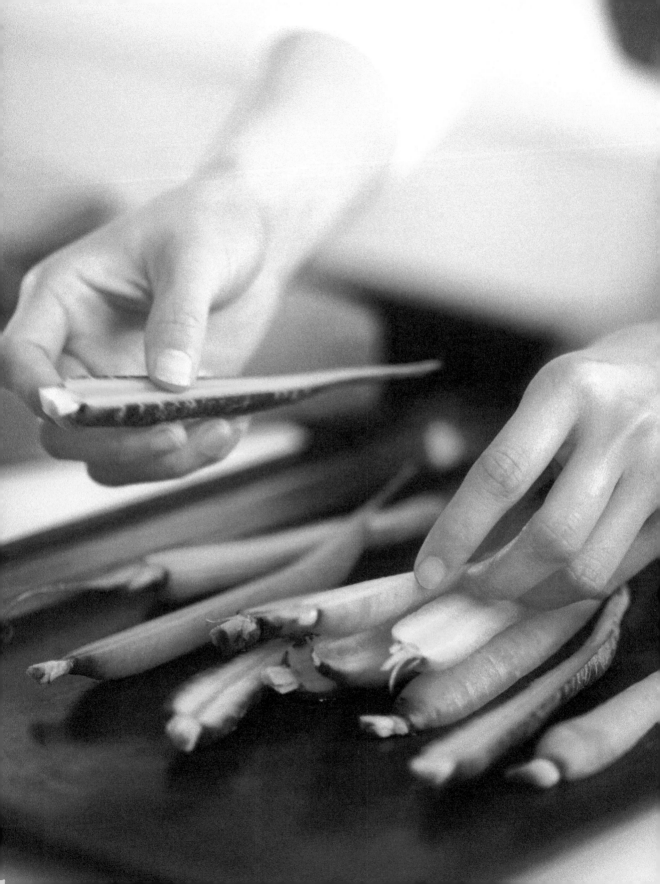

# The Dirty Dozen & The Clean Fifteen

A nonprofit environmental watchdog organization called Environmental Working Group (EWG) looks at data supplied by the US Department of Agriculture (USDA) and the Food and Drug Administration (FDA) about pesticide residues. Each year it compiles a list of the best and worst pesticide loads found in commercial crops. You can use these lists to decide which fruits and vegetables to buy organic to minimize your exposure to pesticides and which produce is considered safe enough to buy conventionally. This does not mean they are pesticide-free, though, so wash these fruits and vegetables thoroughly.

These lists change every year, so make sure you look up the most recent one before you fill your shopping cart. You'll find the most recent lists, as well as a guide to pesticides in produce, at EWG.org/FoodNews.

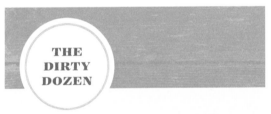

**THE DIRTY DOZEN**

Apples
Celery
Cherries
Cherry tomatoes
Cucumbers
Grapes
Nectarines
Peaches
Spinach
Strawberries
Sweet bell peppers
Tomatoes

*In addition to the Dirty Dozen, the EWG added two types of produce contaminated with highly toxic organophosphate insecticides:*

Kale/Collard greens
Hot peppers

**THE CLEAN FIFTEEN**

Asparagus
Avocados
Cabbage
Cantaloupe
Cauliflower
Eggplant
Grapefruit
Honeydew melon

Kiwis
Mangos
Onions
Papayas
Pineapples
Sweet corn
Sweet peas (frozen)

# Measurement Conversions

## Volume Equivalents (Liquid)

| US STANDARD | US STANDARD (OUNCES) | METRIC (APPROXIMATE) |
|---|---|---|
| 2 tablespoons | 1 fl. oz. | 30 mL |
| ¼ cup | 2 fl. oz. | 60 mL |
| ½ cup | 4 fl. oz. | 120 mL |
| 1 cup | 8 fl. oz. | 240 mL |
| 1 ½ cups | 12 fl. oz. | 355 mL |
| 2 cups or 1 pint | 16 fl. oz. | 475 mL |
| 4 cups or 1 quart | 32 fl. oz. | 1 L |
| 1 gallon | 128 fl. oz. | 4 L |

## Oven Temperatures

| FAHRENHEIT | CELSIUS (APPROXIMATE) |
|---|---|
| 250°F | 120°C |
| 300°F | 150°C |
| 325°F | 165°C |
| 350°F | 180°C |
| 375°F | 190°C |
| 400°F | 200°C |
| 425°F | 220°C |
| 450°F | 230°C |

## Volume Equivalents (Dry)

| US STANDARD | METRIC (APPROXIMATE) |
|---|---|
| ⅛ teaspoon | 0.5 mL |
| ¼ teaspoon | 1 mL |
| ½ teaspoon | 2 mL |
| ¾ teaspoon | 4 mL |
| 1 teaspoon | 5 mL |
| 1 tablespoon | 15 mL |
| ¼ cup | 59 mL |
| ⅓ cup | 79 mL |
| ½ cup | 118 mL |
| ⅔ cup | 156 mL |
| ¾ cup | 177 mL |
| 1 cup | 235 mL |
| 2 cups or 1 pint | 475 mL |
| 3 cups | 700 mL |
| 4 cups or 1 quart | 1 L |

## Weight Equivalents

| US STANDARD | METRIC (APPROXIMATE) |
|---|---|
| ½ ounce | 15 g |
| 1 ounce | 30 g |
| 2 ounces | 60 g |
| 4 ounces | 115 g |
| 8 ounces | 225 g |
| 12 ounces | 340 g |
| 16 ounces or 1 pound | 455 g |

# References

American Heart Association, The. High Blood Pressure. Accessed March 29, 2017. www.heart.org/HEARTORG/Conditions /HighBloodPressure/High-Blood -Pressure-or-Hypertension_UCM_002020 _SubHomePage.jsp.

American Heart Association, The. Nutrition. Accessed March 30, 2017. www.heart.org/HEARTORG/Healthy Living/HealthyEating/Nutrition/Nutrition _UCM_310436_SubHomePage.jsp.

Centers for Disease Control and Prevention. Heart Disease. Accessed March 29 and April 10, 2017. www.cdc.gov/heartdisease.

DASH Eating Plan. National Heart, Lung, and Blood Institute. Accessed March 29, 2017. www.nhlbi.nih.gov/health/health -topics/topics/dash.

Eckel, R. H., Jakicic J. M., Ard J. D., Hubbard V. S., de Jesus J. M., et al. "2013 AHA/ACC Guidelines on Lifestyle Management to Reduce Cardiovascular Risk." *Circulation* (2013): doi.org/10.1161 /01.cir.0000437740.48606.d1.

Harvard T.H. Chan School of Public Health. "Healthy Dietary Styles." *The Nutrition Source.* Accessed March 29, 2017. www.hsph.harvard.edu/nutritionsource /healthy-dietary-styles.

Health.gov. "2015–2020 Dietary Guidelines for Americans." Accessed March 29, 2017. www.health.gov/dietaryguidelines/2015.

University of Maryland Medical Center. Heart Healthy and DASH Diet. Accessed March 30, 2017. www.umm.edu/health /medical/reports/articles/hearthealthy -diet.

*U.S. News & World Reports.* "Best Diets Rankings." Accessed March 28, 2017. http://health.usnews.com/best-diets -overall.

World's Healthiest Foods. Accessed March 30, 2017. www.whfoods.com.

# Resources

MayoClinic.com: This website provides an in-depth description of the DASH diet as well as a two-day sample DASH-diet menu:

- "DASH Diet: Healthy Eating to Lower Your Blood Pressure." www.mayoclinic .org/healthy-lifestyle/nutrition-and -healthy-eating/in-depth/dash-diet /art-20048456.

- "Sample Menus for the DASH diet." www.mayoclinic.org/healthy-lifestyle /nutrition-and-healthy-eating/in-depth /dash-diet/art-20047110?pg=1.

The National Heart, Lung, and Blood Institute (NHLBI) is the creator of the DASH diet, and on their website you will find pages of useful information:

- "DASH Eating Plan." National Heart, Lung, and Blood Institute. www.nhlbi .nih.gov/health/health-topics/topics /dash.

The USDA Dietary Guidelines for Americans recommends the DASH eating plan as a healthy eating pattern to follow. On this site you will find information on food groups, food group servings, and related healthy lifestyle information:

- Health.gov. "2015–2020 Dietary Guidelines for Americans." health.gov/dietaryguidelines/2015.

The Academy of Nutrition and Dietetics website has articles and nutrition information for consumers on heart and cardiovascular health:

- "Heart and Cardiovascular Health." www.eatright.org/resources/health /wellness/heart-and-cardiovascular -health.

The Mediterranean diet shares many similarities to the DASH diet. To learn more visit:

- Mayo Clinic. "Mediterranean Diet: A Heart-Healthy Eating Plan." www.mayo clinic.org/healthy-lifestyle/nutrition -and-healthy-eating/in-depth/mediter ranean-diet/art-20047801.

For a description of symptoms, heart healthy guidelines, and other tools, visit:

- SecondsCount.org. "Nutrition, Diet & Your Health." www.secondscount.org /healthy-living/heart-healthy-nutrition -diet#.WDtIAqIrJ-U.

The American Heart Association website has heart-healthy recipes and nutrition information geared toward the consumer:

- Simple Cooking and Recipes. http://recipes.heart.org/?gclid =CObGs4HsydACFYM2gQodtaoIrA.

- Nutrition. www.heart.org/HEARTORG /HealthyLiving/HealthyEating /Nutrition/Nutrition_UCM_310436 _SubHomePage.jsp.

The Oregon Dairy Council website has a wealth of resources, recipes, and tools to help you get started on following the DASH diet:

- www.dashdietoregon.org.

To find economical recipe ingredients check your local Walmart, Kroger, Safeway, or H-E-B.

# Recipe Index

## A

Apple-Cinnamon Baked Pork Chops, 52, 111
Avocado and Egg Toast, 63

## B

Baked Chickpea-and-Rosemary Omelet, 31, 87
Baked Cod Packets with Broccoli and Squash, 104
Baked Eggs in Avocado, 76
Balsamic-Roasted Chicken Breasts, 50, 97
Banana-Cashew Cream Mousse, 37, 135
Beef-and-Bean Chili, 118
Black-Bean and Vegetable Burrito, 75
Black-Bean Soup, 79
Black-Eyed Peas and Greens Power Salad, 82
Blueberry-Oatmeal Muffin in a Mug, 70
Broccoli with Garlic and Lemon, 125
Brown-Rice Pilaf, 126
Butternut-Squash Macaroni and Cheese, 83

## C

Cantaloupe Smoothie, 71
Carrot-Cake Smoothie, 36, 131
Cauliflower Mashed "Potatoes," 123
Chicken and Broccoli Stir-Fry, 92
Chilled Cucumber-and-Avocado Soup with Dill, 88
Chocolate Cake in a Mug, 133
Chunky Black-Bean Dip, 54, 127
Cilantro-Lime Tilapia Tacos, 101
Classic Hummus, 128
Cranberry Sauce, 38, 145
Creamy Avocado "Alfredo" Sauce, 142
Crispy Almond Chicken, 107
Crispy Potato Skins, 129

## E

Easy Chickpea Veggie Burgers, 89
Easy Cinnamon Baked Apples, 132
Easy Roast Salmon with Roasted Asparagus, 32, 99

## F

Fresh Vegetable Salsa, 56, 147

## G

Garlic Salmon and Snap Peas in Foil, 105
Glazed Grilled Pork Ribs with Honey, Ginger, and
    Soy Sauce, 119
Greek Yogurt Mayonnaise, 39, 146
Grilled Chicken, Avocado, and Apple Salad, 95
Grilled Steak, Onions, and Mushrooms, 53, 117

## H

Healthy Vegetable Fried Rice, 85
Hearty Lentil Soup, 78
Honey-Mustard Chicken, 94

## L

Lemon-Parsley Baked Flounder and Brussels
    Sprouts, 33, 102
Loaded Baked Sweet Potatoes, 80

## M

Make-Ahead Fruit and Yogurt Parfait, 69
Microwave Quiche in a Mug, 28, 62
Mustard-Crusted Pork Tenderloin, 34, 110

## O

Open-Faced Turkey Burger, 98
Orange-Beef Stir-Fry, 35, 115
Overnight Oats with Bananas and Walnuts, 46, 64

## P

Pan-Seared Scallops, 103
Pasta with Tomatoes and Peas, 84
Peach and Blueberry Tart, 136
Peaches and Greens Smoothie, 29, 66
Peanut Butter and Banana Smoothie, 68
Peanut Butter Banana "Ice Cream," 134

Pork Medallions with Spring Succotash, 112
Pork Salad with Walnuts and Peaches, 113
Pork, White Bean, and Spinach Soup, 114
Portobello-Mushroom Cheeseburgers, 86

## Q

Quick Chicken Fajitas, 93
Quick Chicken Stock, 141

## R

Red Beans and Rice, 48, 77
Red Pepper Pesto, 144
Roasted Brussels Sprouts, 124
Roasted Chickpeas, 55, 130

## S

Salmon, Spinach, and Tomato Lasagna, 106
Shrimp Pasta Primavera, 51, 100

Southwestern Bean-and-Pepper Salad, 122
Southwest Tofu Scramble, 30, 74
Spiced Pepper Relish, 57, 149
Sriracha Parsnip Fries, 137
Steak Tacos, 116
Steel-Cut Oats with Blueberries and Almonds, 65
Strawberry Yogurt Smoothie, 47, 67
Super Simple Vegetable Broth, 140

## T

Tangy Barbecue Sauce, 148
Tomato-Basil Sauce, 143
Turkey Cutlets with Herbs, 96

## W

White Beans with Spinach and Pan-Roasted
    Tomatoes, 49, 81

# Index

## A

Alcohol consumption, 2–3, 7
Almonds
    Steel-Cut Oats with Blueberries and Almonds, 65
Apples
    Apple-Cinnamon Baked Pork Chops, 52, 111
    Easy Cinnamon Baked Apples, 132
    Grilled Chicken, Avocado, and Apple Salad, 95
    Make-Ahead Fruit and Yogurt Parfait, 69
Asparagus
    Easy Roast Salmon with Roasted
        Asparagus, 32, 99
Avocados
    Avocado and Egg Toast, 63
    Baked Eggs in Avocado, 76
    Chilled Cucumber-and-Avocado Soup
        with Dill, 88
    Cilantro-Lime Tilapia Tacos, 101
    Creamy Avocado "Alfredo" Sauce, 142
    Grilled Chicken, Avocado, and Apple Salad, 95
    Portobello-Mushroom Cheeseburgers, 86
    Southwestern Bean-and-Pepper Salad, 122

## B

Bananas
    Banana-Cashew Cream Mousse, 37, 135
    Cantaloupe Smoothie, 71
    Carrot-Cake Smoothie, 36, 131
    Overnight Oats with Bananas and
        Walnuts, 46, 64
    Peanut Butter and Banana Smoothie, 68
    Peanut Butter Banana "Ice Cream," 134
    Strawberry Yogurt Smoothie, 47, 67
Basil
    Creamy Avocado "Alfredo" Sauce, 142
    Pan-Seared Scallops, 103
    Pasta with Tomatoes and Peas, 84
    Red Pepper Pesto, 144
    Tomato-Basil Sauce, 143

Beans and legumes. *See also specific*
    Baked Chickpea-and-Rosemary Omelet, 31, 87
    Beef-and-Bean Chili, 118
    Black-Bean Soup, 79
    Black-Bean and Vegetable Burrito, 75
    Chunky Black-Bean Dip, 54, 127
    Easy Chickpea and Veggie Burgers, 89
    Healthy Vegetable Fried Rice, 85
    Hearty Lentil Soup, 78
    Pork Medallions with Spring Succotash, 112
    Pork, White Bean, and Spinach Soup, 114
    Red Beans and Rice, 48, 77
    Southwestern Bean-and-Pepper Salad, 122
    White Beans with Spinach and Pan-Roasted
        Tomatoes, 49, 81
Beef
    Beef-and-Bean Chili, 118
    Grilled Steak, Onions, and Mushrooms, 53, 117
    Orange-Beef Stir-Fry, 35, 115
    Steak Tacos, 116
Bell peppers
    Black-Bean and Vegetable Burrito, 75
    Fresh Vegetable Salsa, 56, 147
    Loaded Baked Sweet Potatoes, 80
    Quick Chicken Fajitas, 93
    Red Pepper Pesto, 144
    Southwestern Bean-and-Pepper Salad, 122
    Spiced Pepper Relish, 57, 149
    Steak Tacos, 116
Berries. *See specific*
Beverages, 7
Black beans
    Black-Bean and Vegetable Burrito, 75
    Black-Bean Soup, 79
    Chunky Black-Bean Dip, 54, 127
Black-eyed peas
    Black-Eyed Peas and Greens Power Salad, 82
Blood pressure, 2
Blood sugar, 8

Blueberries
    Blueberry-Oatmeal Muffin in a Mug, 70
    Peach and Blueberry Tart, 136
    Steel-Cut Oats with Blueberries and Almonds, 65
Broccoli
    Baked Cod Packets with Broccoli and
        Squash, 104
    Broccoli with Garlic and Lemon, 125
    Chicken and Broccoli Stir-Fry, 92
    Quick Chicken Fajitas, 94
Brussels sprouts
    Lemon-Parsley Baked Flounder and Brussels
        Sprouts, 33, 102
    Roasted Brussels Sprouts, 124
Budget-saver recipes
    about, 59
    Avocado and Egg Toast, 63
    Baked Chickpea-and-Rosemary Omelet, 31, 87
    Baked Eggs in Avocado, 76
    Black-Bean Soup, 79
    Black-Eyed Peas and Greens Power Salad, 82
    Blueberry-Oatmeal Muffin in a Mug, 70
    Broccoli with Garlic and Lemon, 125
    Brown-Rice Pilaf, 126
    Cantaloupe Smoothie, 71
    Carrot-Cake Smoothie, 36, 131
    Cauliflower Mashed "Potatoes," 123
    Chicken and Broccoli Stir-Fry, 92
    Chocolate Cake in a Mug, 133
    Chunky Black-Bean Dip, 54, 127
    Classic Hummus, 128
    Cranberry Sauce, 38, 145
    Creamy Avocado "Alfredo" Sauce, 142
    Crispy Almond Chicken, 107
    Crispy Potato Skins, 129
    Easy Chickpea Veggie Burgers, 89
    Easy Cinnamon Baked Apples, 132
    Greek Yogurt Mayonnaise, 39, 146
    Healthy Vegetable Fried Rice, 85

    Hearty Lentil Soup, 78
    Make-Ahead Fruit and Yogurt Parfait, 69
    Microwave Quiche in a Mug, 28, 62
    Open-Faced Turkey Burger, 98
    Overnight Oats with Bananas and
        Walnuts, 46, 64
    Pasta with Tomatoes and Peas, 84
    Peaches and Greens Smoothie, 29, 66
    Peanut Butter and Banana Smoothie, 68
    Peanut Butter Banana "Ice Cream," 134
    Portobello-Mushroom Cheeseburgers, 86
    Quick Chicken Fajitas, 93
    Red Beans and Rice, 48, 77
    Roasted Brussels Sprouts, 124
    Roasted Chickpeas, 55, 130
    Southwestern Bean-and-Pepper Salad, 122
    Spiced Pepper Relish, 57, 149
    Sriracha Parsnip Fries, 137
    Steel-Cut Oats with Blueberries and Almonds, 65
    Strawberry Yogurt Smoothie, 47, 67
    Tangy Barbecue Sauce, 148
    Tomato-Basil Sauce, 143
    Turkey Cutlets with Herbs, 96
    White Beans with Spinach and Pan-Roasted
        Tomatoes, 49, 81

## C

Cabbage
    Black-Eyed Peas and Greens Power Salad, 82
Cantaloupe
    Cantaloupe Smoothie, 71
Carbohydrates, 8
Cardiovascular exercise, 19
Carrots
    Black-Eyed Peas and Greens Power Salad, 82
    Carrot-Cake Smoothie, 36, 131
    Chicken and Broccoli Stir-Fry, 92
    Hearty Lentil Soup, 78
    Pork Medallions with Spring Succotash, 112

Carrots *(continued)*
Quick Chicken Stock, 141
Super Simple Vegetable Broth, 140
Cashews
Banana-Cashew Cream Mousse, 37, 135
Red Pepper Pesto, 144
Cauliflower
Cauliflower Mashed "Potatoes," 123
Celery
Hearty Lentil Soup, 78
Quick Chicken Stock, 141
Super Simple Vegetable Broth, 140
Cheddar cheese
Butternut-Squash Macaroni and Cheese, 83
Cheese. *See specific*
Chicken
Balsamic-Roasted Chicken Breasts, 50, 97
Chicken and Broccoli Stir-Fry, 92
Crispy Almond Chicken, 107
Grilled Chicken, Avocado, and Apple Salad, 95
Quick Chicken Fajitas, 93, 94
Quick Chicken Stock, 141
Chickpeas
Baked Chickpea-and-Rosemary Omelet, 31, 87
Classic Hummus, 128
Easy Chickpea Veggie Burgers, 89
Loaded Baked Sweet Potatoes, 80
Roasted Chickpeas, 55, 130
Chipotle peppers in adobo sauce
Chunky Black-Bean Dip, 54, 127
Cilantro
Black-Bean Soup, 79
Cilantro-Lime Tilapia Tacos, 101
Circulatory system, 2
Cocoa powder
Chocolate Cake in a Mug, 133
Corn
Pan-Seared Scallops, 103
Southwestern Bean-and-Pepper Salad, 122

Cranberries
Cranberry Sauce, 38, 145
Cucumbers
Chilled Cucumber-and-Avocado Soup with Dill, 88

**D**

Dairy products. *See also specific*
to enjoy/avoid, 4–6
pantry staples, 15
DASH diet
benefits of, 9
beverages, 7
and diabetes, 8
equipment, 16–17
foods to enjoy/avoid, 5
guidelines, 4, 6
meal planning, 17–18
pantry clean-out, 12–13
and physical activity, 18–20
recipe information, 59
recommended servings, 6
shopping for, 13, 15
Week One meal plan, 23–39
Week Two meal plan, 41–57
Diabetes, 8
Diastolic blood pressure, 2
Dietary Approaches to Stop Hypertension. *See* DASH diet
Dill
Chilled Cucumber-and-Avocado Soup with Dill, 88
Salmon, Spinach, and Tomato Lasagna, 106

**E**

Edamame
Healthy Vegetable Fried Rice, 85
Eggs
Avocado and Egg Toast, 63
Baked Chickpea-and-Rosemary Omelet, 31, 87
Baked Eggs in Avocado, 76

Healthy Vegetable Fried Rice, 85

Microwave Quiche in a Mug, 28, 62

Electrolytes, 4

Equipment, 16–18

## F

Fats and oils

to enjoy/avoid, 5–6

pantry staples, 15

Fish

Baked Cod Packets with Broccoli and
Squash, 104

Cilantro-Lime Tilapia Tacos, 101

Easy Roast Salmon with Roasted
Asparagus, 32, 99

Garlic Salmon and Snap Peas in Foil, 105

Lemon-Parsley Baked Flounder and Brussels
Sprouts, 33, 102

Salmon, Spinach, and Tomato Lasagna, 106

Flavonoids, 7

Food processors, 18

Frozen produce, 13

Fruits. *See also specific*

to enjoy/avoid, 4–5

pantry staples, 15

## G

Garbanzo beans. *See* Chickpeas

Ginger

Glazed Grilled Pork Ribs with Honey, Ginger,
and Soy Sauce, 119

Grains

and diabetes, 8

to enjoy/avoid, 4–5

Greek yogurt

Banana-Cashew Cream Mousse, 37, 135

Cantaloupe Smoothie, 71

Carrot-Cake Smoothie, 36, 131

Chilled Cucumber-and-Avocado Soup with Dill, 88

Chunky Black-Bean Dip, 54, 127

Greek Yogurt Mayonnaise, 39, 146

Loaded Baked Sweet Potatoes, 80

Make-Ahead Fruit and Yogurt Parfait, 69

Peaches and Greens Smoothie, 29, 66

Peanut Butter and Banana Smoothie, 68

Salmon, Spinach, and Tomato Lasagna, 106

Strawberry Yogurt Smoothie, 47, 67

## H

High blood pressure. *See* Hypertension

Hypertension

risk factors, 2–3

treatment recommendations, 3

Hypertensive crisis, 2

## I

Immersion blenders, 79

Infused water, 7

## L

Leafy greens. *See also specific*

Black-Eyed Peas and Greens Power Salad, 82

Grilled Chicken, Avocado, and Apple Salad, 95

Peaches and Greens Smoothie, 29, 66

Leeks

Super Simple Vegetable Broth, 140

Lemons and lemon juice

Baked Cod Packets with Broccoli and
Squash, 104

Black-Eyed Peas and Greens Power Salad, 82

Broccoli with Garlic and Lemon, 125

Chilled Cucumber-and-Avocado Soup with Dill, 88

Classic Hummus, 128

Creamy Avocado "Alfredo" Sauce, 142

Garlic Salmon and Snap Peas in Foil, 105

Lemon-Parsley Baked Flounder and Brussels
Sprouts, 33, 102

Peach and Blueberry Tart, 136

Lemons and lemon juice *(continued)*
    Shrimp Pasta Primavera, 51, 100
    Turkey Cutlets with Herbs, 96
    White Beans with Spinach and Pan-Roasted
        Tomatoes, 49, 81
Lentils
    Hearty Lentil Soup, 78
Lifestyle changes, 3, 14–15, 18–20
Lima beans
    Pork Medallions with Spring Succotash, 112
Limes and lime juice
    Avocado and Egg Toast, 63
    Baked Eggs in Avocado, 76
    Cilantro-Lime Tilapia Tacos, 101
    Fresh Vegetable Salsa, 56, 147
    Red Beans and Rice, 48, 77
    Southwestern Bean-and-Pepper Salad, 122
    Steak Tacos, 116

## M

Meal planning
    guidelines, 17–18
    Week One, 23–39
    Week Two, 41–57
Medications, 3
Milk, 7–8
    Blueberry-Oatmeal Muffin in a Mug, 70
    Butternut-Squash Macaroni and Cheese, 83
    Cantaloupe Smoothie, 71
    Carrot-Cake Smoothie, 36, 131
    Chocolate Cake in a Mug, 133
    Make-Ahead Fruit and Yogurt Parfait, 69
    Microwave Quiche in a Mug, 28, 62
    Overnight Oats with Bananas and
        Walnuts, 46, 64
    Peach and Blueberry Tart, 136
    Peaches and Greens Smoothie, 29, 66
    Peanut Butter and Banana Smoothie, 68
    Steel-Cut Oats with Blueberries and Almonds, 65

Strawberry Yogurt Smoothie, 47, 67
Mozzarella cheese
    Salmon, Spinach, and Tomato Lasagna, 106
Mushrooms
    Baked Chickpea-and-Rosemary Omelet, 31, 87
    Grilled Steak, Onions, and Mushrooms, 53, 117
    Open-Faced Turkey Burger, 98
    Portobello-Mushroom Cheeseburgers, 86

## N

Neff, Kristin, 14
Noodles. *See* Pasta
Nutrition labels, 8
Nuts. *See specific*

## O

Oats
    Blueberry-Oatmeal Muffin in a Mug, 70
    Easy Chickpea Veggie Burgers, 89
    Make-Ahead Fruit and Yogurt Parfait, 69
    Overnight Oats with Bananas and
        Walnuts, 46, 64
    Steel-Cut Oats with Blueberries and Almonds, 65
One pot recipes
    about, 59
    Apple-Cinnamon Baked Pork Chops, 52, 111
    Baked Chickpea-and-Rosemary Omelet, 31, 87
    Balsamic-Roasted Chicken Breasts, 50, 97
    Beef-and-Bean Chili, 118
    Black-Bean and Vegetable Burrito, 75
    Black-Bean Soup, 79
    Broccoli with Garlic and Lemon, 125
    Brown-Rice Pilaf, 126
    Cauliflower Mashed "Potatoes," 123
    Chicken and Broccoli Stir-Fry, 92
    Chilled Cucumber-and-Avocado Soup with Dill, 88
    Classic Hummus, 128
    Cranberry Sauce, 38, 145
    Crispy Potato Skins, 129

Easy Roast Salmon with Roasted Asparagus, 32, 99

Fresh Vegetable Salsa, 56, 147

Hearty Lentil Soup, 78

Mustard-Crusted Pork Tenderloin, 34, 110

Orange-Beef Stir-Fry, 35, 115

Pan-Seared Scallops, 103

Pork, White Bean, and Spinach Soup, 114

Pork Salad with Walnuts and Peaches, 113

Quick Chicken Fajitas, 93

Quick Chicken Stock, 141

Roasted Brussels Sprouts, 124

Roasted Chickpeas, 55, 130

Shrimp Pasta Primavera, 51, 100

Southwest Tofu Scramble, 30, 74

Spiced Pepper Relish, 57, 149

Steak Tacos, 116

Super Simple Vegetable Broth, 140

Tomato-Basil Sauce, 143

Turkey Cutlets with Herbs, 96

White Beans with Spinach and Pan-Roasted Tomatoes, 49, 81

Onions

Beef-and-Bean Chili, 118

Black-Bean Soup, 79

Fresh Vegetable Salsa, 56, 147

Grilled Steak, Onions, and Mushrooms, 53, 117

Hearty Lentil Soup, 78

Loaded Baked Sweet Potatoes, 80

Quick Chicken Fajitas, 93

Quick Chicken Stock, 141

Spiced Pepper Relish, 57, 149

Super Simple Vegetable Broth, 140

Oranges and orange juice

Orange-Beef Stir-Fry, 35, 115

Strawberry Yogurt Smoothie, 47, 67

## P

Pantry staples, 13, 15

Parmesan cheese

Baked Chickpea-and-Rosemary Omelet, 31, 87

Pasta with Tomatoes and Peas, 84

Red Pepper Pesto, 144

Shrimp Pasta Primavera, 51, 100

Parsnips

Sriracha Parsnip Fries, 137

Pasta

Butternut-Squash Macaroni and Cheese, 83

Pasta with Tomatoes and Peas, 84

Salmon, Spinach, and Tomato Lasagna, 106

Shrimp Pasta Primavera, 51, 100

Peaches

Peach and Blueberry Tart, 136

Peaches and Greens Smoothie, 29, 66

Pork Salad with Walnuts and Peaches, 113

Peanut butter

Peanut Butter and Banana Smoothie, 68

Peanut Butter Banana "Ice Cream," 134

Peas

Garlic Salmon and Snap Peas in Foil, 105

Pasta with Tomatoes and Peas, 84

Physical activity, 3, 18–20

Pineapple

Carrot-Cake Smoothie, 36, 131

Pinto beans

Southwestern Bean-and-Pepper Salad, 122

Pork

Apple-Cinnamon Baked Pork Chops, 52, 111

Glazed Grilled Pork Ribs with Honey, Ginger, and Soy Sauce, 119

Mustard-Crusted Pork Tenderloin, 34, 110

Pork Medallions with Spring Succotash, 112

Pork Salad with Walnuts and Peaches, 113

Pork, White Bean, and Spinach Soup, 114

Portion sizes, 4, 18
Potatoes. *See also* Sweet potatoes
    Crispy Potato Skins, 129
    Super Simple Vegetable Broth, 140
Processed foods, 12–13
Proteins. *See also* Beef; Chicken; Fish; Pork; Turkey
    to enjoy/avoid, 4–6
    pantry staples, 15

## R

Recommended servings, 6
Red beans
    Red Beans and Rice, 48, 77
Rice
    Brown-Rice Pilaf, 126
    Healthy Vegetable Fried Rice, 85
    Red Beans and Rice, 48, 77

## S

Salt, 6
Scallions
    Brown-Rice Pilaf, 126
Scallops
    Pan-Seared Scallops, 103
Self-care, 14–15, 20
Sheet pan recipes
    about, 59
    Baked Cod Packets with Broccoli and
        Squash, 104
    Garlic Salmon and Snap Peas in Foil, 105
    Sriracha Parsnip Fries, 137
Shopping
    guidelines, 13, 15
    Week One meal plan list, 24–25
    Week Two meal plan list, 42–43
Shrimp
    Shrimp Pasta Primavera, 51, 100
Slow cookers, 17

Smoothies, 29
    Cantaloupe Smoothie, 71
    Carrot-Cake Smoothie, 36, 131
    Peaches and Greens Smoothie, 29, 66
    Peanut Butter and Banana Smoothie, 68
    Strawberry Yogurt Smoothie, 47, 67
Snacking, 20
Sodium, 6, 23, 41
Spinach
    Baked Chickpea-and-Rosemary Omelet, 31, 87
    Black-Eyed Peas and Greens Power Salad, 82
    Easy Chickpea Veggie Burgers, 89
    Microwave Quiche in a Mug, 28, 62
    Open-Faced Turkey Burger, 98
    Peaches and Greens Smoothie, 29, 66
    Pork, White Bean, and Spinach Soup, 114
    Pork Medallions with Spring Succotash, 112
    Pork Salad with Walnuts and Peaches, 113
    Red Beans and Rice, 48, 77
    Salmon, Spinach, and Tomato Lasagna, 106
    Southwest Tofu Scramble, 30, 74
    Turkey Cutlets with Herbs, 96
    White Beans with Spinach and Pan-Roasted
        Tomatoes, 49, 81
Spiralizers, 17
Squash. *See also* Zucchini
    Baked Cod Packets with Broccoli and
        Squash, 104
    Black-Bean and Vegetable Burrito, 75
    Butternut-Squash Macaroni and Cheese, 83
    Fresh Vegetable Salsa, 147
    Pan-Seared Scallops, 103
Sriracha
    Sriracha Parsnip Fries, 137
Strawberries
    Strawberry Yogurt Smoothie, 47, 67
Strength training, 19
Stress-relief, 20
Stretching, 19–20

Sugars, 4, 12

Sweet potatoes
    Loaded Baked Sweet Potatoes, 80

Swiss cheese
    Portobello-Mushroom Cheeseburgers, 86

Systolic blood pressure, 2

## T

Tahini
    Classic Hummus, 128

30-minute recipes
    about, 59
    Avocado and Egg Toast, 63
    Baked Chickpea-and-Rosemary Omelet, 31, 87
    Baked Cod Packets with Broccoli and
        Squash, 104
    Baked Eggs in Avocado, 76
    Beef-and-Bean Chili, 118
    Black-Bean and Vegetable Burrito, 75
    Black-Bean Soup, 79
    Black-Eyed Peas and Greens Power Salad, 82
    Blueberry-Oatmeal Muffin in a Mug, 70
    Broccoli with Garlic and Lemon, 125
    Brown-Rice Pilaf, 126
    Butternut-Squash Macaroni and Cheese, 83
    Cantaloupe Smoothie, 71
    Carrot-Cake Smoothie, 36, 131
    Cauliflower Mashed "Potatoes," 123
    Chicken and Broccoli Stir-Fry, 92
    Chocolate Cake in a Mug, 133
    Chunky Black-Bean Dip, 54, 127
    Cilantro-Lime Tilapia Tacos, 101
    Classic Hummus, 128
    Creamy Avocado "Alfredo" Sauce, 142
    Crispy Potato Skins, 129
    Easy Roast Salmon with Roasted
        Asparagus, 32, 99
    Fresh Vegetable Salsa, 56, 147

Garlic Salmon and Snap Peas in Foil, 105
Greek Yogurt Mayonnaise, 39, 146
Grilled Chicken, Avocado, and Apple Salad, 95
Grilled Steak, Onions, and Mushrooms, 53, 117
Healthy Vegetable Fried Rice, 85
Honey-Mustard Chicken, 94
Lemon-Parsley Baked Flounder and Brussels
    Sprouts, 33, 102
Loaded Baked Sweet Potatoes, 80
Make-Ahead Fruit and Yogurt Parfait, 69
Microwave Quiche in a Mug, 28, 62
Mustard-Crusted Pork Tenderloin, 34, 110
Open-Faced Turkey Burger, 98
Orange-Beef Stir-Fry, 35, 115
Pan-Seared Scallops, 103
Pasta with Tomatoes and Peas, 84
Peaches and Greens Smoothie, 29, 66
Peanut Butter and Banana Smoothie, 68
Peanut Butter Banana "Ice Cream," 134
Pork, White Bean, and Spinach Soup, 114
Pork Medallions with Spring Succotash, 112
Pork Salad with Walnuts and Peaches, 113
Portobello-Mushroom Cheeseburgers, 86
Quick Chicken Fajitas, 93
Red Pepper Pesto, 144
Roasted Brussels Sprouts, 124
Shrimp Pasta Primavera, 51, 100
Southwestern Bean-and-Pepper Salad, 122
Southwest Tofu Scramble, 30, 74
Steak Tacos, 116
Steel-Cut Oats with Blueberries and Almonds, 65
Tangy Barbecue Sauce, 148
Tomato-Basil Sauce, 143
Turkey Cutlets with Herbs, 96
White Beans with Spinach and Pan-Roasted
    Tomatoes, 49, 81

Tofu
    Southwest Tofu Scramble, 30, 74

Tomatoes
    Beef-and-Bean Chili, 118
    Black-Bean and Vegetable Burrito, 75
    Black-Bean Soup, 79
    Cilantro-Lime Tilapia Tacos, 101
    Fresh Vegetable Salsa, 56, 147
    Hearty Lentil Soup, 78
    Open-Faced Turkey Burger, 98
    Pan-Seared Scallops, 103
    Pasta with Tomatoes and Peas, 84
    Pork, White Bean, and Spinach Soup, 114
    Quick Chicken Fajitas, 93
    Tomato-Basil Sauce, 143
    White Beans with Spinach and Pan-Roasted
        Tomatoes, 49, 81
Turkey
    Open-Faced Turkey Burger, 98
    Turkey Cutlets with Herbs, 96

## V

Vegan recipes
    about, 59
    Black-Bean and Vegetable Burrito, 75
    Black-Bean Soup, 79
    Black-Eyed Peas and Greens Power Salad, 82
    Broccoli with Garlic and Lemon, 125
    Cauliflower Mashed "Potatoes," 123
    Classic Hummus, 128
    Cranberry Sauce, 38, 145
    Creamy Avocado "Alfredo" Sauce, 142
    Crispy Potato Skins, 129
    Easy Cinnamon Baked Apples, 132
    Hearty Lentil Soup, 78
    Pasta with Tomatoes and Peas, 84
    Peanut Butter Banana "Ice Cream," 134
    Red Beans and Rice, 48, 77
    Roasted Brussels Sprouts, 124
    Roasted Chickpeas, 55, 130
    Southwestern Bean-and-Pepper Salad, 122

Southwest Tofu Scramble, 30, 74
Spiced Pepper Relish, 57, 149
Super Simple Vegetable Broth, 140
Tomato-Basil Sauce, 143
White Beans with Spinach and Pan-Roasted
    Tomatoes, 49, 81
Vegetables. *See also specific*
    to enjoy/avoid, 4–5
    pantry staples, 15
    steaming, 125
Vegetarian recipes
    about, 59
    Avocado and Egg Toast, 63
    Baked Chickpea-and-Rosemary Omelet, 31, 87
    Baked Eggs in Avocado, 76
    Banana-Cashew Cream Mousse, 37, 135
    Blueberry-Oatmeal Muffin in a Mug, 70
    Brown-Rice Pilaf, 126
    Butternut-Squash Macaroni and Cheese, 83
    Cantaloupe Smoothie, 71
    Carrot-Cake Smoothie, 36, 131
    Chilled Cucumber-and-Avocado Soup
        with Dill, 88
    Chocolate Cake in a Mug, 133
    Chunky Black-Bean Dip, 54, 127
    Easy Chickpea Veggie Burgers, 89
    Fresh Vegetable Salsa, 56, 147
    Greek Yogurt Mayonnaise, 39, 146
    Healthy Vegetable Fried Rice, 85
    Loaded Baked Sweet Potatoes, 80
    Make-Ahead Fruit and Yogurt Parfait, 69
    Microwave Quiche in a Mug, 28, 62
    Overnight Oats with Bananas and
        Walnuts, 46, 64
    Peach and Blueberry Tart, 136
    Peaches and Greens Smoothie, 29, 66
    Peanut Butter and Banana Smoothie, 68
    Portobello-Mushroom Cheeseburgers, 86
    Red Pepper Pesto, 144

Sriracha Parsnip Fries, 137

Steel-Cut Oats with Blueberries and Almonds, 65

Strawberry Yogurt Smoothie, 47, 67

Tangy Barbecue Sauce, 148

## W

Walnuts

Make-Ahead Fruit and Yogurt Parfait, 69

Overnight Oats with Bananas and
Walnuts, 46, 64

Pork Salad with Walnuts and Peaches, 113

Water chestnuts

Chicken and Broccoli Stir-Fry, 92

White beans

Pork, White Bean, and Spinach Soup, 114

White Beans with Spinach and Pan-Roasted
Tomatoes, 49, 81

## Y

Yogurt. *See* Greek yogurt

## Z

Zucchini

Black-Bean and Vegetable Burrito, 75

Fresh Vegetable Salsa, 56, 147

Pan-Seared Scallops, 103

# About the Author

Jennifer Koslo is a Registered Dietitian Nutritionist (RDN), Board Certified Specialist in Sports Dietetics (CSSD), Licensed Dietitian in the state of Texas, and an American Council on Exercise Certified Personal Trainer. A member of the Sports, Cardiovascular, and Wellness Practice Group of the Academy of Nutrition and Dietetics (SCAN), she holds a Doctorate of Philosophy in education and a dual Master's of Science Degree in Exercise Science and Human Nutrition. Jennifer's experience includes almost three years as a Peace Corps fisheries volunteer in Sierra Leone, West Africa; working in clinical nutrition as a cardiac dietitian; as the chronic disease nutritionist for a state health department; as a college professor teaching nutrition and sports nutrition; and as a private-practice dietitian doing one-on-one nutrition counseling. Author of six healthy-eating cookbooks—*The 21-Day Healthy Smoothie Plan, Diabetic Cookbook for Two, Healthy Smoothie Recipe Book, The Alkaline Diet for Beginners, The Insulin Resistance Diet for PCOS,* and *The Heart Healthy Cookbook for Two*—Jennifer continues to teach college-level nutrition and sports nutrition, write, and provide individual nutrition counseling and personal-training services through her online business, Koslo's Nutrition Solutions.

CPSIA information can be obtained
at www.ICGtesting.com
Printed in the USA
BVHW01s1030291017
498829BV00001BA/1/P